Drug Use, Policy, and Management

Drug Use, Policy, and Management

Richard E. Isralowitz and Darwin Telias

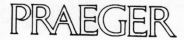

Westport, Connecticut
London

Library of Congress Cataloging-in-Publication Data

Isralowitz, Richard.
   Drug use, policy, and management / Richard E. Isralowitz, Darwin
Telias.
     p. cm.
   Includes bibliographical references and index.
   ISBN 0–275–96128–1 (alk. paper)
   1. Drug abuse—United States. 2. Drug abuse—United States—
Prevention. I. Telias, Darwin, 1939–   . II. Title.
HV5825.I85   1998
363.4′5′0973—DC21   98–14908

British Library Cataloguing in Publication Data is available.

Library of Congress Catalog Card Number: 98–14908
ISBN: 0–275–96128–1

First published in 1998

Praeger Publishers, 88 Post Road West, Westport, CT 06881
An imprint of Greenwood Publishing Group, Inc.

Printed in the United States of America

The paper used in this book complies with the
Permanent Paper Standard issued by the National
Information Standards Organization (Z39.48–1984).

10 9 8 7 6 5 4 3 2 1

Copyright Acknowledgment

The authors and publisher gratefully acknowledge permission to quote from the following:

William Grimes, "The Next to Last Whiff of Smoke and Mirrors," *New York Times*, April 20, 1997.
Copyright © 1997 by The New York Times Co. Reprinted by Permission.

Contents

Preface

Crime and violence, police action and court activity, property confiscation, media attention, massive allocations of federal, state, and local resources, and other factors lead to the conclusion that the drug problem attracts more public concern and attention than any other social issue. Whether illegal substances such as marijuana, heroin, and cocaine or legal substances, including cigarettes and alcohol, drug use is a deeply embedded characteristic of society.

In terms of illegal drugs alone, the U.S. federal government has spent $110,000 million—or $110,000,000,000—over the last ten years to fight the problem. State and local governments are reported to have allocated a comparable amount; and massive sums have been spent by communities, businesses, schools and private individuals attempting to address drug use. "The conservative total from all efforts adds up to close to $500,000 million. This figure does not count the indirect cost of drug use measured in human suffering, increased violence, and lost lives,"[1] nor does it include the damage done by cigarettes and alcohol. Additionally, it has been estimated that illegal drugs have cost more than $300,000 million in health care, incarceration, accidents, and litigation during the 1990s.[2] Such a commitment (i.e., $800,000 million spent over the last ten years) translates to a cost of $29,630 per hard-core addict per year, using the government's estimate that there are about 2.7 million hard-core addicts in America. In terms of U.S. 1997 population census information, nearly $300 per year is being spent on the drug problem for every man, woman, and child in America to convince the public that there is "an abiding willingness on the part of the government and the people to fight back."[3]

The numbers associated with the drug issue are overwhelming, and understanding the extent of the problem is not made any easier by drug policy makers and experts who explain the problem in different, often contradicting, ways. Take for example the statements of government officials and experts that appeared in the same publication issued by the U.S. Information Agency in June, 1997.[4] At that time, Barry McCaffrey (director of the White House National Drug Policy) stated:

[As] a nation we have made enormous progress in our efforts to reduce drug use and its consequences. . . . While America's illegal drug problem remains serious, it does not approach the emergency situation of the late 1970s, when drug abuse skyrocketed, or the cocaine epidemic of the 1980s. In the past 15 years, we have reduced the number of illicit drug users by 50 percent. Just 6 percent of our household population age 12 and over was using drugs in 1995, down from 14.1 percent in 1979. Cocaine use has also plunged, dropping 30 percent in the past four years. More than 1.5 million Americans were current cocaine users in 1995, a 74 percent decline from 5.7 million a decade earlier. Cocaine is on its way out as a major threat in America. In addition, drug-related homicides are down by 25 percent.

In contrast, Mathea Falco (president of Drug Strategies, a nonprofit policy institute in Washington, D.C., who served as a U.S. assistant secretary of state for international narcotics matters from 1977 to 1981) stated:

Two-thirds of the public think that drug abuse is worse today than five years ago. Half say that they know someone who has been addicted to an illegal drug. Since 1980, $290,000 million [has been spent] on federal, state, and local anti-drug efforts. This amount—some $20,000 million a year—is twice as much as the federal government spends annually for all biomedical research, including research on heart disease, cancer and AIDS. . . . Federal policy has been consistent for years: we have spent most of the money trying to reduce the supply of drugs in this country through enforcement, interdiction, and overseas programs to eliminate drug production. Unfortunately, this effort has failed. Despite a fivefold increase in federal expenditures for supply reduction efforts since 1986, cocaine is cheaper today than it was a decade ago. Heroin is sold on the streets for $10 a bag at purities exceeding 60 percent compared to less than 30 percent in 1990. The nation's chief drug enforcement official . . . told Congress in March 1995 that "availability and purity of cocaine and heroin are at an all-time high." And, for the first time, arrests for drug possession reached the one million mark in 1994—a 30 percent increase over the previous three years. . . . Despite America's overseas efforts, worldwide opium and cocaine production has doubled in the last 10 years. The number of countries producing drugs has doubled as well, making drugs a truly global business. . . . Since 1992, adult drug use has gone up 12 percent, the first sustained increase since the 1970s. Among young adults 18–21, one in seven now reports using illegal drugs at least once a month. . . . Marijuana remains the most widely used illegal drug, among both adults and teenagers. . . . Heroin use is increasing, particularly among young professionals and those in the entertainment world. Because of its higher purity, the drug can be snorted or smoked, increasing its appeal to those reluctant to inject drugs. . . . Methamphetamine abuse is also increasing. A synthetic stimulant that produces euphoria, high energy, and self-confidence, the drug may induce violent, paranoid behavior as well as stroke, seizuer, and death. Methamphetamine-related emergency room episodes more than tripled between 1991 and 1994 nationwide. . . . Among medical professionals, the legal narcotic fentanyl—10 times more powerful than heroin—is frequently abused. . . . Mood-altering pharmaceutical drugs [such as Ritalin, which is a central nervous system stimulant;

Rohypnol, which, as a tranquilizer, lowers inhibitions, suppresses short-term memory, and has led to some women being raped by men]; . . . and glue, aerosol sprays, lighter fluid and paint thinner are gaining new popularity . . . and [are being used] by growing numbers of children.

General McCaffrey has reported:

[D]rug education and prevention are the centerpiece of the national drug strategy. . . . [and] diverse drug prevention and education campaigns have been successful. . . . There is no question that effective treatment programs can put people in a position where they no longer suffer from addiction . . . treatment lowers medical costs, reduces accidents and worker absenteeism, diminishes criminal behavior, and cuts down on child abuse and neglect. . . . Unfortunately, there is no cure for addiction, and treatment is often a lifelong undertaking. . . . A 1994 study by the Rand Coproration demonstrated a cost-benefit ratio of seven to one for drug prevention and treatment compared to supply reduction. In other words, for every dollar not spent on drug prevention and treatment, we would have to spend $7 on reducing the supply of drugs. The question is not whether we can afford to pay for treatment. Rather, how can we afford not to?

Falco expressed the belief that

[i]t is doubtful whether any policy to cut off the supply of drugs to America can ever succeed. . . . But if supply cannot be curtailed, perhaps demand can be reduced. Such considerations have led to new interest in drug prevention, treatment, and community efforts to organize citizens against drugs. Yet, most children do not get effective drug prevention teaching, even though such programs can cut new drug use by half. In addition, one million prison inmates in this country have serious drug habits, regardless of the crimes for which they were convicted. Treatment for drug abuse is not readily available inside the criminal justice system or in many communities. Yet, extensive research confirms that treatment is the most cost-effective way to combat addiction and drug-related crime. . . . [Nevertheless], treatment represents less than 20 percent of the nearly 16 billion dollar annual federal budget used for dealing with the drug problem. Serious doubts exist regarding the effectiveness of efforts to combat illegal drugs through law enforcement and military interdiction; yet, approximately 65 percent (approximately $8 billion) of the entire annual drug budget goes for such activity. From an international perspective, $100 million per year is spent by the United States on efforts to control the flow of drugs from Colombia, Bolivia and Peru alone.

For years, efforts to combat the drug problem have been referred to as a "war." Now it appears that there is a retreat from the "war" terminology by government officials. According to General McCaffrey, the metaphor of a "war on drugs" is misleading. It implies a lightning, overwhelming attack. "We defeat an enemy. But who's the enemy in this case? It's our own children. It's fellow employees. The metaphor starts to break down. The United States does not wage war on its own citizens. The chronically addicted must be helped, not defeated. . . . A more appropriate conceptual framework for the drug problem is the metaphor of cancer. Dealing with cancer is a long-term proposition. It requires the mobilization of support mechanisms—human, medical, educational, and societal among others."[5] While the general's remarks raise a number of questions, including the meaning of "war," who the enemy and the victims are, and the use of a medical model approach for defining the drug problem, the important point is that perhaps his words reflect a government shift in terms of how the public is now being led to perceive the drug problem.

Drug policy decision making tends to have taken a roller-coaster ride under the Clinton administration. Beginning with Clinton's first drug administrator, Lee Brown, effort was made to focus drug reform and action on hard-core drug users and addicts and not casual users. With an eye on reelection, however, President Clinton realized that no matter how much new policies were needed to address the drug problem, such revisionist thinking made him vulnerable to Republican attacks that he was soft on drugs and crime. The president's approach to the drug problem shifted back to that of his predecessor but not before Surgeon General Dr. Joycelyn Elders had suggested that she was open to the idea of legalizing or decriminalizing drug possession. Seeing her as expendable and a liability, Clinton terminated her role and abandoned any real effort to make significant changes in U.S. drug policy. Even with the liberalization of marijuana use for "medical" reasons in California and Arizona and the relatively benign nature of that substance compared to cocaine, heroin, alcohol, methamphetamine, a cornucopia of hallucinogens, and other substances, McCaffrey's statement that "we must . . . continue to oppose efforts to legalize marijuana if we want to reduce the rate of teenage drug use and prevent American youth from using more dangerous drugs" tends to be more of a response to the reality of politics rather than the need for realistic policies to address the drug problem.[6]

Without doubt, the most successful achievement in addressing the drug problem does not come from how federal and state governments have dealt with illegal substances but rather their combined efforts to wear down the cigarette industry through litigation. The landmark $360 billion settlement in 1997 has put an end to Joe Camel and the Marlboro Man, cigarette vending machines, and tobacco billboard ads but blocks individual plaintiffs from winning punitive damages from tobacco companies for past actions and collectively limits them to no more than $5 billion annually in compensatory damages. While former surgeon general C. Everett Koop and David Kessler, former head of the Food and Drug Administration, have expressed their reservations about the agreement, there appears to be little argument that the settlement was better than nothing and that the conditions of agreement needed to be resolved quickly because of politics and shifting political fortunes—not only at the state level among attorneys general but at the federal level as well.

With limits on liability in place, cigarette manufacturers including Philip Morris, R. J. Reynolds, and Brown and Williamson, which have banded together to form the U.S. Cigarette Export Association, have moved on to other marketplaces in the world. This is precisely the case for such countries as Japan, Taiwan, and South Korea, where their markets have opened up to U.S. brands and have allowed U.S.

companies a far greater promotional latitude than the state monopolies enjoyed. "The results [have been] dramatic: between 1985 and 1995, the market share of imported cigarettes jumped from 2 to 6 percent in South Korea, 2 to 21 percent in Japan, and zero to 22 percent in Taiwan."[7]

Time is needed to address many of the details of the settlement, but it appears, based on evidence regarding the addictive properties of tobacco, that had it not been for tobacco's legitimate status gained through "big business" tactics and political influence, cigarettes and other tobacco products could have been placed under the rubric of illegal, controlled substances a long time ago. In fact, according to the settlement, nicotine is destined to become regulated in the United States by the Food and Drug Administration as a drug.

Many factors affect drug policy, for example, the determination of whether a substance is legal or illegal and the way drug addiction is addressed in terms of prevention and treatment. The implications regarding such decisions are not simple; in fact, they are so complex that, over time, patterns of control and treatment tend to be reversed.

ABOUT THIS BOOK

Addressing the problem of drug use, regardless of the nature of intervention, may be likened to "craftsmanship." Many skilled drug prevention educators, therapists, counselors, social workers, managers of drug treatment services, and others have acquired and mastered knowledge of the problem and have developed individualized approaches to intervention. There are many others, however, involved with the drug problem, including those coming from perspectives of policy and program decision making as well as those providing individual, group, and family services, who will benefit from the material presented in this book. The materials selected for inclusion have been gleaned from government publications and reports, professional books and journals, and newspaper and magazine accounts, as well as other sources, to present a useful, provocative, and readable book that relates to major stages of the helping process.

This book begins with definitions of key terms commonly used in discussing drugs and drug use: what a drug is and the meanings of use and abuse as well as addiction and dependence—no simple task, because they are used in many different ways in many different settings. Next, the classes of drugs, including cannabinoids, opioids, cocaine, alcohol, amphetamines, methamphetamine, hallucinogenics, and designer drugs, are briefly reviewed. With this background information in place, an examination is given to the social context and reality of drug use. To promote understanding of the importance of this dimension of the drug problem, tobacco is used as a focal point of discussion.

In Chapter 2, our focus shifts to a review of the theoretical considerations and risk factors commonly associated with drug use. Elements of social order; social forces (e.g., environment, values, and morals; interpersonal relations—family and peers; education; and the media); the labeling and criminalization process; and xii Preface

biological and psychological characteristics are summarized. Chapters 3 through 6 describe heroin, alcohol, cocaine, and marijuana, four substances that underpin the drug problem to a major extent, in terms of historical background, and present patterns and trends of use, personality characteristics of those who use the substance, case histories of individuals who have sought treatment, and multination research that provides a cross-cultural perspective of the issue.

An often overlooked aspect of the drug problem is the organization and management of drug services provision. Chapter 7 examines this issue with an overview of the human services perspective, including drug treatment services management. The results of a study of the organization and management of drug service agencies are discussed in terms of developing and managing services with scarce resources, education and training, community outreach services provision for critical target populations, including female and adolescent drug users, treatment and relapse prevention strategies, and research. Finally, the Epilogue to this book reviews the results of the "War Against Drugs" and raises questions about present policies and provides recommendations for future efforts. Appendixes are provided outlining the questions used for two studies reported in the book—patterns and problems of university student alcohol use and the organization and management of drug services agencies.

NOTES

1. Grassley, C. (1997). The U.S. effort to fight drug use. *Focus: Journal of the United States Information Agency* 2, 3 (June): 10.

2. McCaffrey, B. (1997). Dealing with addiction. *Focus: Journal of the United States Information Agency* 2, no. 3, (June): 5.

3. Grassley, C. (1997). The U.S. effort to fight drug use. *Focus: Journal of the United States Information Agency* 2, no. 3 (June): 10.

4. McCaffrey, B. (1997). Dealing with addiction. *Global Issues: Journal of the United States Information Agency* 2, no. 3, (June): 5–9; Falco, M. (1997). Drug prevention makes a difference. *Global Issues: Journal of the United States Information Agency* 2, no. 3 (June): 20–23.

5. McCaffrey, p. 6.

6. Dreyfuss, R. (1997). Hawks and doves: Who's who in the war on drugs. *Rolling Stone*, August 7, p. 42.

7. McGinn, A. (1997). The nicotine cartel. *World Watch*, July/August, p. 22.

Acknowledgments

We, the authors of this book, express our appreciation to our superb editor, Terri Jennings, and our gratitude to our colleagues and students for their constructive feedback on our efforts. Their encouragement and helpful criticism were vital to this effort. We would also like to thank Orli Isralowitz for her review of the chapters and the faculty of Humanities and Social Services, Ben Gurion University, for its support.

Finally, we want to acknowledge the expertise and cooperation demonstrated by our publisher and its employees—specifically our acquisitions editor, Jane Garry, of Greenwood Publishing Group.

Chapter 1

Drug Use and Abuse: Definitions and the Social Context of Reality—Tobacco

TERMS AND DEFINITIONS: AN OVERVIEW

The majority of people have the general idea that they know what a drug is and what addiction is all about. They are wrong. When asked what a drug is they usually mention some characteristics they have heard about, like its being illegal or causing addiction. But not every drug is illegal—for example, alcohol and tobacco are legal in most countries—and not every drug causes addiction. LSD, for example, is generally not considered addictive. Even the word "addiction," has to be clarified. For the most part, it has been substituted by the term "dependence," which refers to (1) a behavioral syndrome, also known as "psychological dependence," and (2) a "physical" or "physiological" dependence. Furthermore, there is a tendency in the professional literature to avoid defining the term "drug"; rather, the preference is to speak about psychoactive substances with reference to classifications and names. For example, the *Diagnostic and Statistical Manual of Mental Disorders* (DSM—4th Edition) of the American Psychiatric Association (1994) lists 11 classes of pharmacological agents: alcohol, amphetamines or similarly acting agents, caffeine, cannabis, cocaine, hallucinogens, inhalants, nicotine, opiates, phencyclidine (PCP) or similar agents, and sedatives, hypnotics, and anxiolytics. There is a 12th residual category for everything else, including anabolic steroids, and nitrous oxide. Even after reading the list carefully, the meaning of "drug" is still not known.

The reason for the lack of a clear definition is that almost anything may be a drug. What makes a substance a drug is not its chemical properties but how it is used by people. A typical example of this is the use and abuse of medications such as substituting an abused opiate substance like heroin with methadone, a controlled opiate substance. Methadone, dispensed in 100 cc. bottles, contains 40 mgs. of the active substance. If a doctor prescribes 30 mgs. of methadone a day for a patient, then 75 cc. are needed from the bottle. If the patient drinks the entire contents of the bottle (100 cc.) instead of the prescribed 75 cc., the addict has ingested 40 mgs. of methadone instead of 30 mgs. The first 30 mgs. were medically and legally prescribed; however, were the other 10 mgs. taken illegally?

Morphine, when used in a hospital by a doctor to treat a patient, is a valuable medication against pain. But if the same ampoule of morphine was stolen from the hospital and used by somebody who is not a physician, the substance may be considered an illegal drug. If the same ampoule of morphine was used by the same doctor in the same hospital not as a medication against pain but because someone, say an opiate addict, paid him to inject the substance, then the doctor may be considered a "drug dealer" subject to being imprisoned and/or having his medical license revoked.

It is commonly believed that laws exist covering every substance considered to be a drug. Indeed, there are international agreements among many countries, like the Geneva Convention, that ban the use of certain substances except for purposes such as medical and experimental research. Such agreements, however, are subject to laws and means of enforcement that vary from country to country. Heroin, for example, may be used by those addicted to the substance for maintenance purposes in some countries but not in others. Cannabis oil may be used medically in the United States but not in many other countries. Other substances may be used on a country-by-country basis, for example, khat in Yemen and cocaine in Peru and Bolivia. The use of alcohol is permitted in most countries, but not all—Saudi Arabia and other Muslim-dominated countries have very strict laws prohibiting its use.

Other substances present complicated legal problems because of their chemical composition. One such example is the illegal hallucinogenic substance popularly called LSD, which in chemical terms is LSD 25 because it is the 25th of the possible 32 derivatives of lysergic acid. If someone sells or uses LSD 26, instead of LSD 25, which has been the case, that person may be well within the law since there is no law prohibiting the use of LSD 26. Another "legal" problem is the amount of substance possessed or used. Some laws permit the possession of a determinate amount of marijuana (usually up to one ounce or 28 grams) or at least consider the violation a minor offense and not a crime like drug dealing. Other legal systems, depending on the country, consider all possessions of an illegal substance, regardless of the amount, a crime. Still others make a distinction between "for one's own use" and for "dealing." Consequently, even the term "legal" has to be defined on a country-by-country as well as a situation-by-situation basis.

The status of substances is not dependent solely on legal considerations. Laboratory analysis may be needed to determine whether a substance is known and has been categorized for response. Drug producers and dealers have come to realize that by modifying certain illegal substances they may avoid legal prosecution for a year or two until the new substance is proven to be harmful or at least determined to be illegal. Consequently, they tend to stay ahead of the laboratories and law by continuously producing new substances.

The meaning of the word "drug" often varies with the context in which it is used. Because terms such as "drug," "drug dependence," "drug abuse," and "drug addiction" are used so often and in so many different ways—varying across geographic locations, from country to country, and changing over time in response to social and economic pressures—it is often difficult to provide accurate, up-to-date definitions of the terms. In the *Guide to Drug Abuse Research Terminology* published in 1982 by the National Institute of Drug Abuse in the United States, nearly three pages were used on these three terms without providing a simple definition for any of them.[1]

From a strictly scientific viewpoint, "a drug is any substance other than food which by its chemical nature affects the structure and function of the living organism.[2] From a sociological perspective, the concept of "drug" is a cultural artifact, a social fabrication, something that has been arbitrarily defined by certain segments of society as a drug.[3] Clearly, society determines what a drug is, and this social definition influences our values, attitudes, and behavior toward substances, whether of a licit or illicit nature. In a sense, therefore, the definition of a drug lies in the subjective realm. In a study conducted in the United States, substances such as heroin, cocaine, marijuana, amphetamines, and barbiturates were regarded by the public as drugs.[4] Psychoactive substances such as alcohol and tobacco are generally not regarded as drugs at all. In neither public law nor public discussion is alcohol regarded as a drug.[5] At present, however, few experts in the drug field would argue that alcohol is not a drug.[6] More than a decade ago, in the early 1970s, tobacco received some attention as a narcotic substance, but it is now widely recognized as being one of the most harmful drugs in use.[7] In 1988 the surgeon general of the United States, C. Everett Koop, stated that all of the criteria used to define addiction are met by tobacco.[8] Yet, a spokesman for the Tobacco Institute in the United States has stated flatly that the claim to tobacco's addictive properties "contradicts common sense."[9]

In sum, a drug may be legal or illegal, harmful or helpful (as is the case of those substances used in medical therapy, such as penicillin). For purposes of this book, the term "drug" refers to those substances having psychoactive properties that influence the mental functioning of humans and consequently have a physical effect on the body as well. Or, a "drug" is a substance used without medical advice in order to improve mood.

Use/Abuse

The terms "drug use" and "drug abuse" are often applied interchangeably; for example, the use of an illegal drug may be considered an abuse. For many people who use marijuana on occasion in order to achieve a state of euphoria, pleasure, or relaxation it may be argued that they do not abuse the substance. Other perspectives of abuse rely on the notion of potential or actual harm. The use of almost any drug, even those under the guidance of a physician, has at least some potential for harm.[10]

The American Medical Association once referred to "abuse" as the use of a drug outside a medical context. Used in this sense, "abuse" conveyed the impression that a behavior is measurable and announced to the world that the nonmedical taking of drugs was undesirable.[11] In 1973, the National Commission on Marijuana and Drug Abuse stated that the term "drug abuse" must be deleted from official pronouncements and public policy dialogue. "The term has no functional utility and has become no more than an arbitrary code word for that drug use which is presently considered wrong. Continued use of this term, with its emotional overtones, will serve only to perpetuate confused public attitudes about drug-using behavior."[11] More than 20 years later, however, it has been found useful to differentiate users and abusers: "Users are those individuals who have tried or continue to use alcohol or other drugs but who are not dependent or addicted. They also fall into different subgroups: a) those who have tried a substance but have discontinued use; b) those who use infrequently and primarily in response to social circumstances; and, c) those who use periodically but infrequently enough to avoid dependence or addictions. . . . Abusers are heavily involved in alcohol or drug use, while level of abuse may range from early dependence to life-threatening use; treatment is clearly the appropriate intervention."[12]

A more recent definition of substance abuse is presented by the American Psychiatric Association:

The essential feature of "substance abuse" is a maladaptive pattern of substance use manifested by recurrent and significant adverse consequences related to the repeated use of substances. There may be repeated failure to fulfill major role obligations, repeated use in situations in which it is physically hazardous, multiple legal problems, and recurrent social and interpersonal problems. . . . Unlike the criteria for "substance dependence," the criteria for "substance abuse" do not include tolerance, withdrawal, or a pattern of compulsive use and instead include only the harmful consequences of repeated use. . . . Although a diagnosis of "substance abuse" is more likely in individuals who have only recently started taking the substance, some individuals continue to have substance-related adverse social consequences over a long period of time without developing evidence of "substance dependence." The category of "substance abuse" does not apply to caffeine and nicotine.[13]

Addiction/Dependence

It has been known for at least 2,000 years that certain drugs "have the power to enslave men's minds," but it was not until the nineteenth century that the nature of physical addiction or dependence began to be understood. At that time a classic definition of the problem was being developed based on the opiates—at first opium and morphine, and then, after the turn of the century, heroin as well. "Much later, it was recognized [that] alcohol, sedatives, such as barbiturates, and minor tranquilizers also produced most of the symptoms of 'classic' addiction."[14]

Classic addiction or dependence is understood to mean that when a person takes certain drugs in "sufficient quantity over a sufficiently long period of time, and stops taking them abruptly, the user will experience a set of physical symptoms known as withdrawal," which are likely to include chills, fever, diarrhea, muscular twitching, nausea, vomiting, cramps, and general body aches and pains, especially in the bones and joints.[15] Yet not all drugs, even when used over time and in large quantities, produce withdrawal symptoms when the substance is discontinued. Therefore, not all drugs fit the "classic" definition of addiction.

According to the *Diagnostic and Statistical Manual of Mental Disorders* (DSM—4th Edition), the essential feature of "substance dependence" is a cluster of cognitive, behavioral, and physiological symptoms indicating that the individual continues use of the substance despite significant substance-related problems. There is a pattern of repeated self-administration that usually results in tolerance, withdrawal, and compulsive drug-taking behavior. These important terms are defined as follows:

Tolerance is the need for greatly increased amounts of the substance to achieve intoxication (or the desired effect) or a markedly diminished effect with continued use of the same amount of the substance. The degree to which tolerance develops varies greatly across substances. Individuals with heavy use of opiates and stimulants can develop substantial (e.g., tenfold) levels of tolerance, often to a dosage that would be lethal to a nonuser. Alcohol tolerance can also be pronounced, but is usually much less extreme than for amphetamines. Many individuals who smoke cigarettes consume more than 20 cigarettes a day, an amount that would have produced symptoms of toxicity when they first started smoking. Individuals with heavy use of cannabis are generally not aware of having developed tolerance. . . . It is uncertain whether any tolerance develops to phencyclidine (PCP).

Withdrawal is a maladaptive behavioral change, with physiological and cognitive concomitants, that occurs when blood or tissue concentrations of a substance decline in an individual who had maintained prolonged heavy use of the substance. After developing unpleasant withdrawal symptoms, the person is likely to take the substance to relieve or to avoid those symptoms, typically using the substance throughout the day beginning soon after awakening. Withdrawal symptoms vary greatly across the classes of substances. . . . Marked and generally easily measured physiological signs of withdrawal are common with alcohol, opiates, and sedatives, hypnotics, and anxiolytics. Withdrawal signs and symptoms are often present, but may be less apparent, with stimulants such as amphetamines and cocaine, as well as nicotine. No significant withdrawal is seen even after repeated use of hallucinogens.

Dependence or compulsive drug-taking behavior is when an individual takes the substance in larger amounts or over a longer period than was originally intended (e.g., continuing to drink until severely intoxicated despite having set a limit of only one drink). The individual may express a persistent desire to cut down or regulate substance use. Often, there have been many unsuccessful efforts to decrease or discontinue use. The individual may spend a great deal of time obtaining the substance, using the substance, or recovering from its effects. In some instances of *Substance Dependence*, virtually all of the person's daily activities revolve around the substance. Important social, occupational, or recreational activities may be given up or reduced because of substance use. The individual may withdraw from family activities and hobbies in order to use the substance in private or to spend more time with substance-using friends.[16]

According to the World Health Organization, dependence syndrome is a

cluster of physiological, behavioral, and cognitive phenomena in which the use of a substance or a class of substances takes on a much higher priority for a given individual than other behaviors that once had greater value. A central descriptive characteristic of the dependence syndrome is the desire [often strong, sometimes overpowering] to take psychoactive drugs [which may or may not have been medically prescribed] including alcohol or tobacco. There may be evidence that return to substance use after a period of abstinence leads to a more rapid reappearance of other features of the syndrome than occurs with nondependent individuals. . . . It is an essential characteristic of the dependence syndrome that either psychoactive substance taking or a desire to take a particular substance should be present; the subjective awareness of compulsion to use drugs is most commonly seen during attempts to stop or control substance use. . . . The dependence syndrome may be present for a specific substance (e.g., tobacco or diazepam), for a class of substances (e.g., opioid drugs), or for a wider range of different substances (as for those individuals who feel a sense of compulsion regularly to use whatever drugs are available and who show distress, agitation, and/or physical signs of a withdrawal state upon abstinence).[17]

THE CLASSES OF DRUGS: A REVIEW

Alcohol

Alcohol, like heroin, cocaine, and LSD, is a psychoactive substance. Alcohol is "addictive." It generates severe withdrawal symptoms when the heavy, long-term drinker discontinues its use. In fact, alcoholism is by far the most common form of drug addiction, except for tobacco. In the United States, it is estimated that there are 10 million alcoholics and only half a million heroin addicts.[18]

The magnitude of alcohol use and problems associated with its use have been overshadowed in recent years by the preoccupation with the widespread use of drugs such as cocaine and crack, as well as the threat of AIDS, but "[t]ake the deaths from every other abused drug . . . add them together, and they still don't equal the deaths or the cost to society of alcohol alone."[19] In the United States alone:

[a]lcoholism claims tens of thousands of lives each year, ruins untold numbers of families, and costs $117 billion a year in everything from medical bills to lost work days. . . . Cirrhosis of the liver kills at least 14,000 alcoholics a year. Drunk drivers [tend to cause] about half of the annual driving fatalities [which in 1986 totaled 43,000 deaths]. Alcohol was implicated in up to 70% of the 4,000 drowning deaths [in 1986] and in about 30% of the nearly 30,000 suicides . . . nearly a third of the nation's 523,000 state prison inmates drank heavily before committing rape, burglaries and assaults. As many as 45% of the country's more than 250,000 homeless are alcoholics.[20]

Patterns of alcohol use can range from occasional episodes to daily heavy drinking. Dependence can vary from periodic use that cannot be controlled, moderated, or stopped to physical dependence that cannot be stopped without significant and dangerous withdrawal. Indications of alcohol use include a sedated, intoxicated appearance and alcohol odor. Physical addiction to alcohol is characterized by a need to maintain alcohol to prevent physical withdrawal. Abrupt discontinuation of alcohol can be dangerous in cases of physical addiction necessitating medical supervision.

Opiates

This class of drugs includes opium and its derivatives, including substances such as codeine, morphine, heroin, and methadone. Inclusive of this category may be artificial substances, labeled "opioids," with the property to interact with opiate receptors in the brain. Opiate-based substances calm users; however, they have the potential of producing an initial state of euphoria. The substances may be eaten, but they are generally smoked, sniffed, or injected subcutaneously or intravenously. The subcutaneous injection, referred to as "skin-popping," produces a slower absorption with a lower degree of euphoria but longer-lasting effects including characteristic marks on the skin. Addiction to opiates is rather quick, generally after one or two months of daily use. People under the influence of opiates appear calm, sometimes sleepy, and have a tendency to take everything in stride. The situation changes radically when the first symptoms of withdrawal appear, generally six to eight hours after the last use.

Pure opiates cause relatively little body damage; however, those substances sold on the streets as "opiates" usually contain a large amount of contaminants, including poison, which can produce serious damage or even death to the user. Unlike stimulants, opiates do not produce a psychotic state when used in their pure form and have the ability to reduce or eliminate psychotic symptoms in mental patients.

Stimulants

Stimulants such as cocaine, crack, and methamphetamine produce an increased state of arousal accompanied by a sense of confidence and euphoria. Users tend to appear in a state of hyperactivity, agitation, or exhaustion; and, when used over prolonged periods of time, irrational and paranoid behavior may be evidenced. Other characteristics may include regular episodes of out-of control use despite increasing negative consequences associated with that pattern of behavior, weight loss, numerous needle marks, and hyperactivity, as well as problems with work and interpersonal relations. Stimulants can be snorted, injected, smoked, or eaten. When used with heroin, the combination is referred to as "speedball."

Considerable attention is being given to methamphetamine, even small amounts of which can produce euphoria, enhanced wakefulness, increased physical activity, decreased appetite, and increased respiration. Among the effects on the central nervous system are irritability, insomnia, confusion, tremors, anxiety, aggression, and convulsions. A synthetic drug, methamphetamine is related chemically to amphetamine but produces greater effect on the central nervous system. It is reported that the euphoric effects are similar to, but last longer than, those of cocaine. Also, the substance is cheaper to obtain than cocaine.[21]

Methamphetamine was used by soldiers to help them fight off fatigue during World War II, and immediately after the war, with the availability of military surplus, the substance became widely used in Japan. "In the United States in the 1950's, legally manufactured tablets of methamphetamine were used nonmedically by college students, truck drivers, and athletes, who usually did not become severely addicted. This pattern changed drastically in the 1960's with the increased availability of injectable methamphetamine. . . . [The substance] has been the most prevalent clandestinely produced controlled substance in the United States since 1979."[22] Its production is easy and cheap. "Setting up a lab to produce a substantial amount of the drug may cost less than $2,000 and be enormously profitable—one day's production may be worth $70,000."[23]

A structurally similar substance to methamphetamine and the hallucinogen mescaline is "ecstasy." A synthetic drug, ecstasy has been used increasingly among young adults as well as college and high school students. According to the National Institute of Drug Abuse's (NIDA) 1996 Monitoring the Future study, nearly 5 percent of 10th and 12th graders and about 2 percent of 8th graders said they had used ecstasy in the past year.[24] Like methamphetamine, ecstasy has been linked to long-term brain damage that remains long after the high has worn off.[25]

Sedatives, Hypnotics, and Tranquilizers

This class of drugs is commonly known as "downers." They are usually prescription drugs used to reduce anxiety or facilitate sleep. When abused, they induce a sedated, intoxicated state that may eventually result in sleep. The most commonly abused drugs in this class are the benzodiazepines (Valium, Xanax, Ativan, Halcion, Dalmane, Restoril, and others), barbiturates (Phenobarbital, Seconal, Nembutal, Fiornal, Tuinal), and sleeping pills (Placidyl, Doriden, and Quaaludes—which are no longer legally available in the United States through a prescription—and chloralhydrate). All are normally taken in pill form, but they can sometimes be injected. Indications of sedative and hypnotic use include an intoxicated appearance without the odor of alcohol and, in some cases, complaints of anxiety and insomnia. Addiction to sedative and hypnotic drugs is similar to opiate addiction in that there is a physical addiction resulting in a need to maintain enough of the drug in the body to avoid physical withdrawal. The consequences of an abrupt discontinuation of these drugs can be a life-threatening withdrawal syndrome, including seizures. Medical intervention is always necessary in a case of addiction to any of these drugs.

Marijuana and Other Hallucinogens

Hallucinogens include marijuana, hashish (hash), lysergic acid diethylamide (LSD), peyote, and mushrooms. The detrimental effects related to the use of these drugs range from addiction to impaired functioning, cognitive impairment, and reduced motivation. Among the indications of use are bloodshot eyes, unusual behavior, and expressions of bizarre ideas. The habitual user of marijuana or hashish will experience a withdrawal syndrome characterized by roughly 30 days of irritability, insomnia, and craving for the substance upon its discontinuation.

PCP and "Designer Drugs"

PCP (phencyclidine, angel dust, sherms) affects the user at different times as a stimulant, a hallucinogen, an analgesic, or a sedative. Although the strange hallucinogenic effects accompanied by violence are most commonly reported by the media, the PCP addict usually reports effects and behavior patterns similar to those using stimulants. PCP can be snorted, smoked, eaten, or injected. Since it is fat-soluble, it takes a prolonged period to leave the body. Designer drugs are synthetically manufactured substances that mimic other drugs.[26]

THE SOCIAL CONTEXT AND REALITY OF DRUG USE

The use of illicit drugs, alcohol, and other addictive substances is not a new phenomenon but one that takes on meaning and importance in relation to its social context, which varies over time and geographic location. Social context is a powerful determinant of what the drug is and does to the user; it influences at least four central aspects of the drug reality—drug definitions, drug effects, drug-related behavior, and the drug experience. The history of the drug and its use, the social strata of society that use it, the kinds of situations in which it is used, and the publicity and public opinion about it may all be included in the definition of a drug's social context. "How a drug is regarded—by the public, the law, its users, and even the medical profession—depends as much on irrational cultural factors as on its objective properties."[27]

Tobacco

Tobacco is a leafy plant, a stimulant, indigenous to North, Central, and South America. It provides insight of how social context affects the reality of substance use. Introduced to Columbus by natives of the New World, the substance found its way to Europe, and its importance was closely tied to economic interests. The Spanish, for example, had a monopoly on tobacco sales for over 100 years until the British colonies, notably Virginia, were able to produce sufficient quantities from the seventeenth century onward. Tobacco use has taken the form of cigarette, cigar, and pipe smoking, snuff, and chewing. In the United States, Native Americans had long cultivated tobacco and used it in various forms. During the colonial period of the seventeenth century, tobacco was an important cash crop, and it was a federally taxed commodity that was used to help finance the Civil War. By the 1890s, cigarette machines were perfected and greatly increased production. Consumption increased dramatically between 1900 and the mid-1960s.[28]

Use of tobacco, a psychoactive drug, is one of the major causes of debility and premature death in developed countries. Midway into the nineteenth century and long before authentic scientific evidence emerged about the extent of the health risks they posed, cigarettes were labeled "coffin nails."[29] In 1963, cigarette use in the United States reached an all-time high, precipitating the 1964 surgeon general's report that definitively linked cigarette smoking to health problems.[30] In 1980, the surgeon general said that cigarette smoking is the single most important preventable cause of death and disease. Among the key arguments against cigarette use have been that (1) smoking is a major cause of coronary heart disease for both men and women; (2) the risk of developing coronary heart disease and dying from it grows with increasing exposure to smoking, as measured by how deeply one inhales, the age at which one starts, the years one has smoked, and the number of cigarettes smoked per day. Overall, the death rate from coronary heart disease is 70 percent higher among cigarette smokers than among nonsmokers; those who consume two or more packs per day incur two to three times the risk; (3) smoking acts synergistically with other risk factors—principally, elevated cholesterol levels and hypertension; (4) women who smoke and use oral contraceptives have a risk of heart attack that is approximately tenfold higher than that of women who neither smoke nor use oral contraceptives; and (5) smokers have a two- to fourfold risk of sudden death, as compared with nonsmokers.[31]

In 1988 additional facts revealed that cigarettes and other forms of tobacco are addicting, that nicotine is the drug in tobacco that causes addiction, and that pharmacological and behavioral processes that determine addiction are similar to those that determine addiction to drugs such as heroin and cocaine.[32] Moreover, there appears to be a link between cigarette smoking and illegal drug use; for example, adolescents who smoke are more likely to progress to marijuana, cocaine, and heroin than nonsmokers.[33]

In 1989, the U.S. surgeon general reported the following: smoking was the third leading cause of death in the United States; by 1986 lung cancer had caught up with breast cancer as the leading cause of cancer death in women; gender differences in smoking behavior were disappearing; smoking was associated with cancer of the uterine cervix; 43 chemicals in tobacco smoke were determined to be carcinogenic; approximately 390,000 deaths per year were attributable to smoking; disparities in smoking prevalence, quitting, and initiation between groups with the highest and lowest levels of educational attainment were substantial; and educational attainment appeared to be the best single sociodemographic predictor of smoking. Also, there was recognition that prevention and cessation interventions needed to target specific populations with a high smoking prevalence or at high risk of smoking-related disease. These populations included minority groups, pregnant women, military personnel, high school dropouts, blue-collar workers, unemployed persons, and heavy smokers. Regarding youth, one-quarter of high school seniors who ever smoked had their first cigarette by the sixth grade; one-half by the eighth grade. There was a growing body of evidence that economic incentives such as excise taxation of tobacco products, workplace financial incentives, and insurance premium differentials for smokers and nonsmokers affected health behavior, particularly in terms of discouraging the use of tobacco products. While over 50 million Americans continued to smoke, it was reported that more than 90 million would have been smoking if there were no changes in the smoking and health environment since 1964.[34]

From an environmental perspective, findings on cigarette smoking revealed that nonsmokers can be seriously affected from the smoke of cigarettes used by others. Drawing upon 50 studies, the Environmental Protection Agency concluded that "passive smoking" not only aggravates 1 million existing cases of childhood asthma each year but causes 8,000 to 26,000 new cases. Also, it was found that environmental tobacco smoke is linked to pneumonia, bronchitis, and reduced lung function as well as middle-ear effusion, a leading ailment requiring childhood surgery. It has been estimated that every year environmental tobacco smoke causes about 3,000 lung cancer deaths.[35]

Economic Considerations

The modern history of tobacco reflects a population of users from all levels of society, the rich as well as the poor. Its production and sales have represented big business for hundreds of years, not only for growers and manufacturers but for governments in the form of tax revenues. In the United States in 1987, it was estimated that about $4.8 billion per year in taxes to the federal government were generated, and an equal amount of tobacco tax revenues filled state coffers. It has been pointed out that at a time when its trade deficit is of concern, the billions of dollars' worth of cigarettes exported by the United States is not an insignificant factor.[36] The tobacco industry estimates that it directly generates over $40 billion of the gross national product and provides employment for over 700,000 people.[37] Additionally, it has been reported that between $12 and $35 billion is spent each year in the United States alone to treat smoking-related diseases—a significant revenue source for health-related services and industries.[38] According to a 1992 Price Waterhouse report, the tobacco industry was responsible, directly or indirectly, for the employment of about 2.3 million Americans in 1990, including 426,000 employed by the industry, 225,000 employed by its suppliers, and 1.6 million supported by their salaries. Price Waterhouse estimated that the tobacco industry and its suppliers generate about $10.6 billion in federal taxes and $8.3 billion in state and local taxes each year.[39]

Tobacco has secured its position in many societies by controlling the behavior of its consumers through vigorous marketing methods (e.g., the introduction of filter cigarettes in the 1950s, low-tar cigarettes in the 1960s, and then smokeless and perfumed cigarettes) as well as by commanding a special position among governmental policymakers, who for years have protected the substance for reasons beyond the "best interests" of the public.

The glamour era of cigarette advertising . . . began soon after World War I, when American servicemen picked up the cigarette habit. Tobacco executives [claimed] that their wares not only tasted wonderful but claimed that they soothed jangled nerves, prevented weight gain and aided digestion. . . . In the 1920's, Lucky Strike introduced the slogan "Reach for a Lucky Instead of a Sweet" using celebrity endorsers like George M. Cohan, Amelia Earhart and Helen Hayes to bring the message home. The fight-fat campaign made a giant stride toward capturing a new market of female smokers, already primed by the daring Chesterfield campaign that showed a male smoker and his sweetheart spooning under—what else?—a June moon. "Blow Some My Way," the caption read. Well into the 1950's, cigarette advertisers continued to proclaim the health benefits of their product. "How are your nerves?" an ad for one brand asked and proposed a test. Any man who could not button a vest in 12 seconds probably suffered from frayed nerves and should begin smoking immediately. Camels announced that its special Turkish tobacco stimulated the flow of digestive fluids and raised the level of alkalinity in the stomach. Kool, in the brand's early days, even claimed to offer protection against catching colds. For anyone with medical doubts, the tobacco industry wheeled out legions of unnamed doctors who were absolutely sold on the merits of cigarette smoking, or the virtues of one brand. "More doctors smoke Camels than any other cigarette," one ad proclaimed. . . . From the outset, cigarette makers relied on athletes, movie stars and newsmakers to lend luster to their product. Even before World War I, cigarette packs came with cards featuring baseball players and boxers. In the 1950's Ronald Reagan, as an actor, lent his magic touch to Chesterfields, a brand endorsed by Joe Lewis in 1947 as "the champ of cigarettes." . . . The word chutzpah acquired new meaning when Newport unrolled its "Alive With Pleasure" campaign. One ad showed a group of beautiful young achievers playing a fast-action game of beach volleyball, cigarettes still clenched between their teeth. . . . No one expects a cigarette company to portray the typical customer fighting for breath after climbing a flight of stairs, but the cheerful association of cigarettes with youth, energy and athletic excellence has persisted through the decades, mind bogglingly unchanged. . . . As the century turns, though, no athlete or movie star would get within a mile of a Camel advertisement.[40]

During the last few years, however, there has been a reversal of tobacco industry fortunes led by a vigorous campaign against the substance by the Food and Drug Administration in the United States and the medical community. Report after report reveals collusion and manipulation by tobacco companies to promote and preserve a market for their product, including special populations such as children and youth, women, and minority people. Reports such as "Children and Tobacco: The Problem," "Relationship between Cigarette Smoking and Other Unhealthy Behaviors among our Nation's Youth: United States," "Current Trends in Cigarette Advertising and Marketing," "Nicotine Addiction in Young People," "Looking through a Keyhole at the Tobacco Industry," "Nicotine and Addiction," "Lawyer Control of Internal Scientific Research to Protect Against Products Liability Lawsuits," "Lawyer Control of the Tobacco Industry's External Research Program," "Environmental Tobacco Smoke," "The Brown and Williamson Documents," and others have paved the way for a tidal wave of litigation and legislation restricting advertising and the sale of cigarettes and other tobacco products in the United States.[41]

Cigarette companies have been accused of manipulating cigarette nicotine:

Whether by sprayed-on additives, or selection and blend of the leaf or by filters and ventilation devices, cigarette makers have tinkered with their nicotine and tar content since before the first Surgeon General's report in 1964. Indeed, the National Cancer Institute, presumably as a public service, spent more than $50 million from 1968 to 1978 toward developing a less hazardous cigarette by manipulating the toxic yield of tobacco smoke. As the evidence about smoking [mounted], the F.D.A. [U.S. Food and Drug Administration] or Congress could at any time have put a lid on toxic ingredients in cigarettes, as the manufacturers themselves might have done. What we have witnessed instead is a protracted exercise of avoidance by all parties.[42]

In response to a *New York Times* editorial by Anna Quindlen, "Where There's Smoke" (March 2, 1994) the chairman and chief executive officer of R. J. Reynolds Tobacco Company, James W. Johnston, and the president and chief executive officer of Philip Morris, USA, William I. Campbell, summed up the position of the cigarette companies by stating that "cigarettes are a legal product, and more than 50 million American adults choose to smoke. We are proud of the quality standards in making our product."[43]

By all accounts, cigarette smoking is on the decline, particularly in the United States, Western Europe, and other countries despite vigorous marketing attempts as a result of public opinion and politically responsive government. Nevertheless, with people in Western countries already addicted, tobacco industries have focused their efforts on other countries like those in Asia, Eastern Europe, the former Soviet Union, Latin America, and Africa for new profits. While many governments in Asia have launched antismoking campaigns, their efforts have been overwhelmed by the "Madison Avenue glitz" unleashed by the major cigarette companies. Several Asian nations have banned cigarette advertising on television and radio in recent years; but the tobacco companies often find ways around the bans through indirect promotions that skirt the law—sports events, glossy advertisements for clothing brands or travel agencies that bear the name and logo of a cigarette brand. With 1.2 billion people and the world's fastest growing economy, for example, China is a primary target of multinational tobacco companies, and "physicians say that the health implications of the tobacco boom in Asia are nothing less than terrifying, and there are frequent comparisons here to the Opium War of the mid-19th century when the British went to war to force the Chinese to accept imports of a dangerous addictive drug—opium, an important cash crop for British merchants."[44]

CONCLUSION

Examination of tobacco reveals the relationship between the viewpoint of a dominant group and the social context within which it arises. The patterns of response over time regarding tobacco products, particularly cigarettes, reflect the shifting patterns of policy toward the use of a harmful substance. Clearly, the tobacco industry built an impenetrable infrastructure that remained a bulwark for years against challenges to their products no matter how harmful to the health of individuals and their families. Reasons why this substance has, to a large extent, until the present, remained relatively unscathed or immune lie in the realm of economics and politics.

People's consciousness of drug use and abuse, manifested through attitudes and behavior, appears to be determined by their social being at a particular time and in a particular physical setting. The basis of this thinking is not new; it is the fundamental proposition of the sociology of knowledge, which includes the concepts of ideology (ideas serving as weapons of social interests) and false consciousness. To understand the meaning of drug use and abuse among people, it is helpful to be concerned with everything that passes for knowledge in society. "As soon as one states this, one realizes that the focus on intellectual history is ill-chosen, or rather, is ill-chosen if it becomes the central focus of the sociology of knowledge. Theoretical thought, 'ideas,' are not that important in understanding the drug issue, since they are only a small part of what passes as 'knowledge.' What must be addressed is what people know as reality in their everyday lives."[45]

For tobacco, a guardian of the social order decided what was permissible to use. The dos and don'ts of drug use are defined by the purveyors of society, who include moralists, entrepreneurs, politicians, law enforcers, and others. Wars have been waged in order to preserve the social construction of "drug" reality, the two most notable being the Opium Wars in the nineteenth century and the present "war on drugs" being fought by many countries. It would be naive to think of the drug problem in only economic terms, the profits made legally through sales taxes, health remedies and treatments, prevention programs, jobs, and so on, and illegally through the manufacturing, marketing, and sale of illicit substances. But it would be equally naive to ignore this powerful factor and its role in shaping how and which drugs are provided and used throughout the world.

NOTES

1. Ray, E., and Ksir, C. (1990). *Drugs, Society and Human Behavior.* St. Louis: Times Mirror/Mosby, p. 4.

2. National Commission on Marijuana and Drug Abuse (1973). *Drug use in America: Problem in perspective. Second report of the NCMDA.* Washington, DC: U.S. Government Printing Office, p. 9.

3. Goode, E. (1989). *Drugs in American Society.* 3rd ed. New York: McGraw-Hill, p. 23.

4. Abelson, H., Cohen, R., Schrayer, D., and Rappaport, M. (1973). *Drug Experience, Attitudes, and Related Behavior among Adolescents and Adults, Part 1.* Princeton, NJ: Response Analysis.

5. National Commission on Marijuana and Drug Abuse, p. 10.

6. Ray and Ksir; Johnston, L., O'Malley, P., and Bachman, J. (1987). *National Trends in Drug Use and Related Factors among American High School Students and Young Adults, 1975–1986.* Rockville, MD: National Institute on Drug Abuse.

7. Brecher, E. (1972). *Licit and Illicit Drugs.* Boston: Little, Brown, p. 223; Goode, p. 210.

8. Goode, p. 211.

9. Tolchin, M. (1988). Surgeon general asserts smoking is an addiction. *New York Times,* May 17, p. A1; Goode, p. 211.

10. Ray and Ksir, p. 4.

11. Goode, pp. 25–26.

12. National Commission on Marijuana and Drug Abuse, p. 13; Lorion, R., Bussell, D., and Goldberg, R. (1991). Identification of youth at high risk for alcohol or other drug problems. In E. Goplerud (ed.), *Preventing Adolescent Drug Use: From Theory to Practice.* OSAP, DHHS Pub. No. (ADM) 91-1725. Washington, DC: U.S. Government Printing Office.

13. American Psychiatric Association (1994). *Diagnostic and Statistical Manual of Mental Disorders.* 4th ed., Washington, DC: American Psychiatric Association, p. 182.

14. Goode, p. 46.

15. Ibid.

16. American Psychiatric Association, pp. 176–178.

17. World Health Organization (1992). *The ICD-10 Classification of Mental and Behavioural Disorders: Clinical Descriptions and Diagnostic Guidelines.* Geneva: World Health Organization, pp. 72–77.

18. Goode, p. 108.

19. Desmond, E. (1987). Out in the open: Changing attitudes and new research give fresh hope to alcoholics. *Time Magazine,* November 30, p. 29.

20. Ibid., pp. 29–30.

21. National Institute of Drug Abuse (1996). Facts about Methamphetamine. *NIDA Notes,* November/December.

22. National Institute of Drug Abuse (1997). Methamphetamine abuse. *NIDA Capsules,*(C-89-06), October.

23. U.S. Department of Justice (1992). *Drugs, Crime, and the JusticeSystem.* A National Report from the Bureau of Justice Statistics. Washington, DC: U.S. Government Printing Office, p. 41.

24. National Institute of Drug Abuse (NIDA). (1997). Study takes a closer look at "Ecstasy Use." *NIDA Notes,* March/April.

25. Mathias, R. (1996). Like methamphetamine, "ecstacy" may cause long-term brain Damage. *NIDA Notes,* November/December; Fischer, C., Hatzidimitriou, G., Wlos, J., Katz, J., and Ricaurte, G. (1995). Reorganization of ascending 5-HT axon projections in animals previously exposed to recreational drug 3,4-methelenedioxymetham-phetamine (MDMA, "ecstasy"). *Journal of Neuroscience* 15: 5476–5485.

26. McCann, M., Rawson, R., Obert, J., and Hasson, A. (1994). *Treatment of Opiate Addiction with Methadone.* Rockville, MD: U.S. Department of Health and Human Services, pp. 28–31.

27. Goode, p. 16.

28. Horgan, C. (1993). *Substance Abuse: The Nation's Number One Health Problem.* Princeton, NJ: Robert Wood Johnson Foundation.

29. Kluger, R. (1996). A peace plan for the cigarette wars. *New York Times Magazine,* April 7, p. 28.

30. Goode, p. 211.

31. U.S. Surgeon General (1982). *The Health Consequences of Smoking for Cancer.* DHHS Publication No. (PHS) 82-50179. Washington, DC: U.S. Government Printing Office; U.S. Surgeon General (1983). *The Health Consequences of Smoking; Cardiovascu-*

lar Disease. DHHS Publication No. (PHS) 84-50204. Washington, DC: U.S. Government Printing Office.

32. U.S. Surgeon General (1988). *The Health Consequences of Smoking: Nicotine Addiction.* DHHS Publication No. (CDC) 88-8406. Washington, DC: U.S. Government Printing Office.

33. Goode, p. 204.

34. Koop, C. (1989). *Reducing the Health Consequences of Smoking—25 Years of Progress: A Report of the Surgeon General.* Rockville, MD: U.S. Department of Health and Human Services.

35. Cowley, G. (1992). Poison at home and at work. *Newsweek,* June 29, p. 49.

36. Shannon, I. (1989). World cigarette pushers. *New York Times,* (IE) August 20, p. 6.

37. Ray and Ksir, p. 203.

38. Molotsky, I. (1985). Smokers' ills cost billions, U.S. says. *New York Times,* September 16, p. A13.

39. Sullum, J. (1996). Last drag. *Across the Board,* March, p. 46.

40. Grimes, W. (1997). The next to last whiff of smoke and mirrors. *New York Times,* (IE), April 20, p. 2.

41. Kessler, D. (1995). Sounding board: Nicotine addiction in young people. *The New England Journal of Medicine* 333, no. 3: 186–189; Food and Drug Adminstration Press Office (1995). Children and tobacco: The problem. FDA Press Office release. August 10; Willard, J., and Schoenborn, C. (1995). Relationship between cigarette smoking and other unhealthy behaviors among our nation's youth: United States, 1992. Washington, DC: U.S. Department of Health and Human Services, Centers for Disease Control and Prevention, Number 263, April 24; Davis, R. (1987). Current trends in cigarette advertising and marketing. *The New England Journal of Medicine* 316, no. 12: 725–732; Glantz, S., Barnes, D., Bero, L., Hanauer, P., and Slade, J. (1995). Looking through the keyhole at the tobacco industry: The Brown and Williamson Documents. *The Journal of the American Medical Association,* 274, no. 3: 219–224; Slade, J., Bero, L., Hanauer, P., Barnes, D., and Glantz, S. (1995). Nicotine and addiction: The Brown and Williamson Documents. *The Journal of the American Medical Association* 274, no. 3: 225–233; Hanauer, P., Slade, J., Barnes, D., Bero, L., and Glantz, S. (1995). Lawyer control of internal scientific research to protect against products liability lawsuits: The Brown and Williamson Documents. *The Journal of the American Medical Association* 274, no. 3: 234–240; Bero, L., Barnes, D., Hanauer, P., Slade, J., and Glantz, S. (1995). Lawyer control of the tobacco industry's external research program: The Brown and Williamson Documents. *The Journal of the American Medical Association* 274, no. 3: 241–247; Barnes, D., Hanauer, P., Slade, J., Bero, L., and Glantz, S. (1995). Environmental tobacco smoke: The Brown and Williamson Documents. *The Journal of the American Medical Association* 274, no. 3: 248–253.

42. Kluger, R. (1994). Of course they manipulate cigarette nicotine. *New York Times,* (IE), March 15, p. 6.

43. Campbell, W. (1994). Decrease in levels. *New York Times,* (IE), March 15, p. 6.

44. Shenon, P. (1994). Asia's having one huge nicotine fit. *New York Times,* (IE), May 15, p. 1.

45. Berger, P., and Luckmann, T. (1967). *The Social Construction of Reality.* New York: Doubleday, p. 15.

Chapter 2

Theoretical Considerations and Risk Factors

Drug use and dependence may be explained as a biomedical, psychological and/or sociological phenomenon. A social science approach, however, tends to consider factors that fall into three major theoretical perspectives: (1) society through its policy and decision-making processes (e.g., determining the societal normative order and allocating resources) is a prime force in shaping problems associated with drug use; (2) certain sociological forces shape a person's personality and cause deviant behavior; and (3) those who use and abuse drugs have physical and/or personality characteristics that precipitate involvement with such activity. Additional considerations include (1) the history of drug abuse patterns and the changing population of users; (2) recognition that specific drug abuse patterns are culturally determined—that cultures (and subcultures) differ in the availability of drugs and the extent of abuse; (3) awareness that demographic (and epidemiological) characteristics of abusers depend on the time period, nation, and locale selected for study; (4) the need to delineate the specific drug (or drugs) of abuse, route of administration, and length of dependence; (5) the etiology of social context in which drug abuse begins; (6) the influence of major institutions (e.g., family, community, peer group, schools, and media) upon the onset and continuation of drug dependency; (7) why drug abuse is more prevalent in certain populations than others; and (8) determination of institutional supports that promote successful treatment and rehabilitation, including consideration of how persistent behavior in subcultures can be changed.[1]

The following interrelated sociological and social-psychological factors represent a paradigm for understanding drug use and dependence.

THE SOCIAL ORDER

People are often referred to as deviant when they do not share the values or adhere to the social norms regarding conduct and personal attributes prescribed by society. While the process of identifying deviance involves the use of normative definitions that may vary over time, the essential nature of deviant behavior is that it reflects a departure from the norms of a particular society.

Beginning in the mid-1930s, the principal focus of sociologists was on a systematic analysis of social and cultural sources of deviant behavior in order to discover how some social structures exert pressure upon certain persons in society to engage in nonconformist, rather than conformist conduct.[2] According to Robert Merton, a person's location in the social system offers differential access to societal goals. In this mean/ends schema, deviant behaviors such as those related to drug use represent the individual's rejection of both the culturally prescribed goals and available means of success. For Merton, the rejection and subsequent behavioral manifestations that are deviant may be labeled a form of retreatism.[3] Merton also pointed out that the lack of opportunity was not the only reason for the high frequency of deviant behavior but, rather, that the differences in the level of accessibility of societal goals are, in fact, class-dependent.[4]

Merton's theory, then, is an attempt to account for the distribution of deviant behavior within a social system and for differences in the distribution and rates of deviant behavior among people by functions or system properties (i.e., the ways in which cultural goals and opportunities for realizing them are distributed).[5] This theory has been applied to drug use and abuse,[6] but never successfully. While the original article, which hardly mentions drug addiction or alcohol, is considered a classic of its kind and is "probably the single most cited article in the entire sociological literature," a number of researchers consider the theory inadequate and irrelevant when applied to etiology or causality of drug use, and these days the theory is not given much attention.[7]

With the 1960s came growing signs of dissatisfaction with both the definition of deviance and the explanatory variables. The main thrust of this criticism was the failure of the theory to "regard deviance as a process [by which] persons become labeled deviant and a concern with organizational responses or adaptation to deviance."[8] Perhaps the most serious attempts to redefine the study of deviance came from Erving Goffman and Howard Becker.[9] An example of the shift in thought is found in Becker's definition of deviance that "social groups create deviance by making the rules whose infractions constitute deviance, and by applying those rules to particular people and labeling them as outsiders."[10] Deviance, then, is less a matter of the act a person commits but concerns how those who make the rules—and can enforce them—view the act and/or the person or class of person who has committed it.

While the theories of Merton, Goffman, and Becker contribute, in part, to understanding deviant behavior in the context of drug use, their explanations fail to include the role of personality and its interface with other forces that shape attitudes and behavior that are defined as outside the acceptable social order.

From the 1940's to the 1960's, most of the ethnographic studies in the drug field shifted the emphasis from asking why people used drugs to asking how they went about getting involved in drug use and how they remained involved. Rather than looking for underlying causes, ethnographers began to search for etiological influences in the social world rather than the internal world of experimenters. This period constituted the first major shift away from psychoanalytic theory and a medical model of addiction to a more sociological perspective. . . . Building on the work of Hughes (1959) who introduced the study of occupations into sociology, Becker (1963) took the career model and applied it to deviant careers in general and drug users specifically. This conceptual shift has broad implications and was the basis for what came to be viewed as a new sociological movement called the "labeling theory."[11]

SOCIAL FORCES: PHYSICAL ENVIRONMENT, VALUES, AND MORALS

From research conducted as early as the 1920s in the United States, it has been shown that the environment where a person lives can be an influential factor in the use and abuse of drugs. An environment that is deteriorating and poverty-stricken serves as a breeding ground for such behavior. Living in this type of setting are people from the lower end of the social hierarchy who are usually beset with a huge assortment of personal and family problems. In order to exist, norms and values different from those prescribed through explicit and implicit social policies, rules of governance, and methods of enforcement are adopted by these people, enabling them to achieve goals that are readily attainable and less abstract.[12]

In one of the major examinations of structure theory, Miller[13] contends that deviant behavior is the product of goals and means that are prescribed by, and common to, members of the lower classes. Conflicts between the middle and lower classes are considered irrelevant, since most of the lower classes have little interest in either the goals or methods of the middle class. Miller argues that people at the bottom of the social hierarchy are inured to the cultural and economic deprivations they have to endure and that they have little expectation of reforming their society or bettering their position in it. In order to gain a sense of personal worth and satisfaction, lower-class people need to build their culture around values that can be more readily sustained than those of the middle class. The result is a destructive pattern of goals and practices that can be endorsed by deprived people despite the opposition of those in society supporting the normative order.[14] Based on this theory, drug use may be considered a natural consequence of adherence to a lower-class normative structure and the associated values and morals.

Cohen suggests that lower-class individuals with behavior such as drug use adopt their own system of values and morals in order to maintain self-respect and status while being confronted with the omnipotent judgments of others. He contends that people in institutional settings are constantly being evaluated (e.g., in the school, on the job, under the law, etc.) by representatives of the middle class. Therefore, poor and minority members face handicaps and frustrations when their teachers and other institutional officials discriminate against them and fail to recognize the problems with which they are confronted. Furthermore, Cohen has written that understanding and equal treatment are difficult, especially for institutional workers having middle-class values, middle-class language, and middle-class stereotypes alleging the inferiority of the lower classes. In the case of a drug offender, characteristics such as family status, place of residence, skin color, ethnic affiliation, and the language and habits acquired in early socialization may be perceived (by those judging the offender) as symbols of weakness, immorality, and deviance.[15]

The issue of access and opportunity is another perspective of why certain people adhere to a deviant set of values and morals. Cloward and Ohlin maintain that legitimate and illegitimate methods of achieving social objectives are differentially distributed among the various groups and classes of a society, so that some have access primarily to legitimate means, others to illegitimate ones, and still others to both methods of attaining their goals. This theory focuses on the disparity between what lower-class people are led to want and what is actually available to them. The authors believe that this issue is one of the major factors contributing to problem attitudes and adjustment.[16]

Through their theory, Cloward and Ohlin attempted to portray several delinquent subcultures, one of which was the "retreatist" subculture of addicts, which was based on a theoretical category developed by Merton, Cloward's mentor. The only empirical study that provided actual descriptions of addict behavior and supported this perspective was Finestone's short description in "Cats, Kicks and Color." It became the sole basis of support for a theory that was soon to achieve national prominence [in the United States]. . . . Because of the importance of the Cloward and Ohlin opportunity theory and its use as the underpinning . . . [for delinquency and antipoverty programs], their mini-theory of addicts as double failures within a retreatist subculture became a persistent theme.[17]

While issues such as lower-class values and morals and the disproportionate number of crime and drug problems found among the poor have been widely covered by sociological research and literature, some studies have shown that such problem behavior is also indigenous to the middle and upper classes. For example, Schur discusses the point that there is much more actual problem behavior than is officially recorded. An implication of "hidden crime" is that "in the main it [is] lower-class crime that [is] officially dealt with and middle- and upper-class offenses that [remain] hidden."[18] This becomes clear through self-reports of crime and drug problems taken from samples of the general population. Consistent with this, Short and Nye found that problem behavior was distributed more evenly throughout the socioeconomic structure of society.[19] Basically, those studies that take as their focus the problem of middle- and upper-class deviance point out that reliance on the theories of drug use being a lower-class phenomenon requires closer scrutiny.[20]

By no means does this review of physical environment, values, and morals imply that drug use is a social-class phenomenon. The facts and statistics reveal that drug use and abuse are a problem that transverses all social classes but also tends to be more easily rooted among the poor in conditions that are consistent with poverty and social degradation.

INTERPERSONAL RELATIONS: THE FAMILY

The role of the family is often referred to as a major causal factor in shaping the personality and behavior of children. The family serves as a reference group on personal and normative levels. Ideally, the child should receive sustenance, recognition, approval, and appreciation from family members for participation in those goals held in common. As a normative reference or "bonding" group, members of the family serve as agents of a culture, transmitting norms, attitudes, and values to the child; how long the family remains a reference group for the child may depend on how well it serves his or her needs.[21]

It is the family which is a major transmission belt for the diffusion of cultural standards to the oncoming generation. But what has until lately been overlooked is that the family largely transmits that portion of the culture accessible to the social stratum and groups in which the parents find themselves. It is, therefore, a mechanism for disciplining the child in terms of the cultural goals and mores characteristic of this narrow range of groups. . . . Quite apart from direct admonitions, rewards and punishments, the child is exposed to social prototypes in the witnessed daily behavior and casual conversations of parents.[22]

Parents train their children to conform or not to conform to particular moral standards through the examples they provide by their own behavior. For example, research indicates a greater amount of socially deviant behavior (e.g., drug use, alcoholism, and criminality) in the parents of problematic youth than in the parents of law-abiding children. It has also been found that "the mother's conformity to socially approved modes of conduct [seems] to be a stronger influence for a child's good conduct than the father's behavior; a combination of two socially deviant parents produced the highest crime rates in the children."[23] Investigators of families with a drug-abusing member have identified some consistent patterns related to adolescent drug use, including the theme of a dominant mother who is overindulgent, overprotective, and manipulative and a father who is far more subordinate, being viewed as weak, inept, and uninvolved.[24]

Since Paul Goodman's Growing Up Absurd was published in 1960, it has been common to trace the long series of societal changes that have narrowed down a household to a nuclear unit, then sent mothers into the labor force, and lastly, with increasing divorce rates, further limited a child's opportunity for receiving parenting.[25] In discussing the transition of youth to adulthood, the report of the Panel on

Youth of the President's Science Advisory Committee (1973), for example, mentions that throughout the nineteenth century in America households provided a variety of people from whom the child could draw support and with whom he or she could identify. During that time, the family was dominant, and young persons were introduced as quickly as possible to a work situation to aid the economy of the family. Knowledge, skills, and values acquisition came primarily from the family and church.[26]

In the traditional folk society, the norms were generally simple. There was a limited range of possibilities for human action, so the rules necessary were also limited. Too, the norms tended to be tied together in a "neater" package. Family life, educational life, and economic life were so closely related that they were difficult to separate. The norms that governed a father and son in a field were, at the same time, familially, educationally, and economically important. If the son violated a norm, the negative sanction, i.e., punishment, for this violation would be immediate and certain. The specific deviant act by the son, however, would be considered in terms of his "whole" personality, his total actions, past and present. His behavior would be seen as "bad," but the son would not likely be considered a deviant person because of such an isolated action.[27]

With industrialization and the growth of a technological and urbanized society, family structures and functions have experienced great change. "The family . . . may no longer be the major socializing influence. Rather, that responsibility is shared today with other societal institutions and with peer groups.[28] Broken homes, a mother-present/father-absent or father-weak household structure, inconsistent discipline, abuse, threats, verbal attacks, and other negative familial characteristics have been linked to drug use and dependence.[29] Additionally, research shows that parental divorce, arrest, a lack of closeness between parents and children, parent and sibling drug use, family disorganization, father unemployed, one or both parents missing, a perceived lack of parental support, lack of identification with a positive male figure, family emphasis on independence instead of self-discipline and community responsibility, and mental illness—all correlate with alcohol and drug abuse among young people in the family.[30] The quality of the parent-child relationship; the quality and consistency of family management; family structure; attachment; communication within the family; modeling of substance use; approval and tolerance of substance use; involvement; absence of closeness of parents; low educational aspirations for the children; lack of parental involvement in the child's activities; weak parental control and discipline; death or absence of a parent; and emotional, physical, or sexual abuse are other factors that have been correlated with drug use.[31]

In a study of the family role in fostering or mitigating substance abuse, it has been found that parent-youth relationships influence a young person's use of alcohol and other drugs. Nonusers felt closer to their parents, considered it important to get along with them, and wanted to be like them. The parents of nonusers set more limits, provided more praise and encouragement, and were less likely to use substances themselves.[32] It has also been found that drug addiction correlates to parental rejections, a lack of emotional warmth in the family, and overprotection.[33]

Regarding addicts, the role of the father has been found to be a predictor of narcotic addiction among boys. "The degree of attachment at ages 12–14 to one's father is a major determinant of how strong a young person's resistance will be to the temptations offered by addiction in neighborhoods where high levels of drug abuse are prevalent. . . . A positive home atmosphere and a strong parental commitment are similarly a strong predictor of the addiction history of young people . . . approximately 40% of the population studied came from families without natural parents in the household and the addict subject perceived his father in a negative fashion."[34]

Peers

Peer relations are a factor often linked to drug use and dependence. Such behavior may be learned through association and interaction with others who are already involved with drugs. A person's relationship with peers may serve as a means of providing the individual with an escape from other interpersonal dealings that he wishes to avoid, such as family, school, or work. Interaction with peers may also be a means by which a person can receive emotional gratification, recognition, reinforcement, security, self-protection, and defense for his or her deviant behavior.[35]

Despite much earlier research that points in the direction of peer influences being most prevalent among lower-class persons,[36] Erickson and Empey believe that their data do not support the notion that peer standards have more importance for the lower classes than they do for the middle class.[37] In fact, their findings lead them to hypothesize that because the youth are departing perhaps even further from the expectations of their parents than lower-class children, middle-class drug users have a greater need for peer support than lower-class offenders. In either case, however, the friends of a drug user and commitment to peer values appear to be far more predictive of such problematic behavior than social class. Additional research reveals that a high level of adolescent peer activity predicts marijuana use; the more that adolescents are isolated and alienated from the parental subculture, and the more involved they are with the teenage peer subculture, the greater the likelihood that they will experiment with, and use, drugs; and users tend to be friends of users, and the selective peer group interaction and socialization therefore constitute probably the single-most powerful influence related to drug use among young people.[38] A study of drug consumption (i.e., marijuana, amphetamines, and tranquilizers) among young adults showed this type of behavior to be related to those who share an apartment (flat) with friends and who are in disagreement with their parental upbringing.[39] There tends to be a progression of roughly four stages among young people regarding substance use: (1) beer or wine; (2) cigarettes or hard liquors; (3) marijuana; and (4) other illegal drugs. "Adolescents rarely skip stages; thus drinking alcohol is necessary to smoking marijuana, just as marijuana use is necessary to moving on to more dangerous drugs such as cocaine and heroin."[40] In another study using a four-variable simplex model to prove the progression theory of substance use, it was found that alcohol use predicted marijuana use, and marijuana use predicted hard drug use.[41] Regarding drug abuse patients in treatment in the United States, it was found that onset of heroin addiction for males commonly began as a peer group recreational activity at an early age (14–18 years); for females onset usually started with their addicted boyfriends.[42]

From this review, it may be concluded that "association with substance-using peers . . . is among the strongest predictors of . . . substance use. Peer influence, approval and/or tolerance of substance use, and modeling have been identified as salient variables. Strong bonds to family and school, however, usually decrease the influence of antisocial peers."[43]

Education

The school is a major agent of status definition in society and has established a critical role in the socialization process of people; consequently, it should be considered an important facet of the drug problem. As a social transmission agency, the school has become an institution that labels youth as winners or losers and by doing so frequently determines the directions they take in conducting their lives.

The school system and its personnel may be perceived as an organization which produces, in the course of its activities, a wide variety of careers [including those of an asocial, deviant and problematic nature]. Within the organizational setting of the school, the day-to-day activities of adolescents and personnel define, classify, and process a wide range of "routine" and "problem" behaviors. Because the school occupies a strategic position as a coordinating agency between the activities of the family, the police, and the peer group vis-à-vis adolescents, it serves as a "clearinghouse" which receives and releases information from and to other agencies concerning adolescents.[44]

Many studies have shown a strong relationship between a negative school experience and drug use. For example, negative attitudes toward school, low academic aspirations and educational achievement, and disciplinary problems in school often precede the onset of drug use and/or dropping out of school. Furthermore, teenage pregnancies and frequency of school absenteeism correlate with increasing levels of drug use.[45]

The educational process, the school and its personnel are a potent force for youth in terms of shaping their attitudes and behavior. Too often, however, the full impact of the school's resource base is lost. Communications between teachers and parents, particularly in the areas of strengthening and reinforcing the learning processes of youth during nonschool hours, tend not to be emphasized. Also, school policy and program administrators normally take a system's maintenance approach of the education process rather than one of a developmental nature that draws upon available resources to address the broad spectrum of community needs in terms of programs, especially during evenings, vacation periods, weekends, and summer months. Most important, the school is too often limited in its ability to prepare young people for a rewarding and happy life, one that will help come to grips with the normative structure and demands of their society.

Media

Since the 1920s when motion pictures became a major source of mass entertainment, the effects of the media have been subject to scientific inquiry and public concern.[46] It has long been recognized that movies, television, and popular "hard rock" music portray an excessive amount of violence and illegal behavior. As early as 1954, a Gallup poll found that seven out of ten American adults attributed the postwar rise in problem behavior among youth, at least in part, to the high incidence of criminal acts shown in the media.[47] Crime, as it is portrayed through certain aspects of the media, encourages and causes improper attitudes and behavior among some children. Testimony before a U.S. Senate subcommittee in 1955 reported that television was serving as a preparatory school for antisocial activity.[48] Information presented by the media provides young persons with an awareness of the external world; however, such information, if not qualified, can also enhance the likelihood that they will behave in an inappropriate and lawless manner. The causal connection between media and problem behavior has been the subject of over 1,000 studies, including a surgeon general's special report in 1972[49] and a National Institute of Mental Health report ten years later.[50]

Regarding exposure to media (i.e., television, movies, video games, video cassettes, newspapers, books, comics, radio, CDs, tapes, etc.), "the average adolescent spends roughly eight hours daily in some form of mass media."[51] In a survey of youth it was found that those who listened to more radio and watched more music, videos, cartoons, and soap opera were more likely to engage in behavior such as drinking alcohol, sex, and smoking cigarettes.[52]

In terms of societal beliefs, the mass media shape people's ideas about what the real world is like,[53] what people think about, and which issues they consider most important.[54] From the perspective of individual behavior, a considerable number of experimental studies show that media can teach specific acts of problem behavior even after controlling for the effects of socioeconomic class, education, and race.[55] Also, there is a cumulative effect of the influence of media over an extended period of time.[56] Behavior, such as drug use, in the media can have a lasting effect on children and youth if (1) the themes presented are repeated often enough; and (2) the information imparted by the media is not clearly contradicted by significant others such as parents, peers, or teachers. In fact, lessons learned by children from the media may be supported, either explicitly or implicitly, by the statements and actions of parents. Adults do not always frown on immorality, and the child may observe his parents occasionally approving illegal behavior or hear them condoning someone's violation of the law.[57] "While it may be true that television, movies, comic books, [popular music], etc. will excite antisocial conduct from only a relatively small number of people, we can also say that the heavy dosage of [problem behavior] in the media heightens the probability that someone in the audience will behave [that way] in a later situation."[58]

Despite widespread concern about the effects of the media, particularly violence through television, there has been surprisingly little empirical research on drinking and drug use. What is known is that there are four basic types of television content presenting substance-related stimuli: (1) television commercials centrally feature positive portrayals of beer and wine drinking; (2) public service announcements typically warn against alcohol abuse, drunk driving, and cocaine use; (3) newscasts disseminate information about problematic outcomes of substance misuse, including reports of drunk-driving accidents, drug-related deaths and arrests, and health risks; and (4) entertainment programming, particularly dramas, movies, and comedy shows, frequently portray characters using alcohol and experiencing positive and/or negative consequences; occasional depictions of other drugs are also presented. While substance use and abuse are shaped by a variety of personality characteristics, family and peer influences, and sociodemographic factors, television is also considered to play an influential role.[59]

Many issues need to be examined and questions answered regarding the impact of the media on shaping drug behavior. Nevertheless, it is clear that, to a large extent, drug use has been popularized by the media. For young people needing only a slight stimulus to engage in drug use, there are many sources to be found.

LABELING-CRIMINALIZATION PROCESS

Building on the work of Everett Hughes[60] who introduced the study of occupations into sociology, Howard Becker[61] took the career model and applied it to deviant careers in general and drug users specifically. This conceptual shift has broad implications and was the basis for what came to be viewed as a new sociological movement called the "labeling theory." When applied to the field of addiction, it provided a different perspective that included an analysis of the individual drug users and of public policy, as well as a legal framework within which such activities took place. In this way, Becker's concepts helped structure the way drug ethnographers began to collect and analyze data. The shift in concept was evident in [Becker's] own study, "Becoming a Marijuana User" [published in 1953].[62]

The labeling process is a method that determines the fate of a person. It tends to reinforce problem behavior rather than ameliorate it. Essentially, labeling theories are less interested in the problem behavior of persons and their characteristics than in the criminalization process by which a community seeks out its law violators, stigmatizes them, and assigns them to a negative status. The following assumptions have been suggested by Schrag as best characterizing the labeling-criminalization process:

[N]o act is intrinsically criminal. It is the law that makes an act a crime. Crimes therefore are defined by organized groups having sufficient political power to influence the legislative process; . . . criminal definitions are enforced in the interest of powerful groups by their official representatives, including the police, courts, correctional institutions, and other administrative bodies. While the law provides detailed guidelines in its substantive definitions and rules of procedure, the way the law is implemented may be determined by the decisions of local officials who depend upon political and social leaders for financial support or other resources; . . . a person does not become a criminal by violating the law. Instead, he is designated a criminal by the reactions of authorities who confer upon him the status of an outcast and divest him of some of his social privileges; . . . only a few persons are caught in violation of the law, though many may be equally guilty. The ones who are caught may be singled out for specialized treatment; . . . criminal sanctions . . . vary according to characteristics of the offender; . . . for any given offense, they tend to be most frequent and severe among males, the young, the unemployed or underemployed, the poorly educated, members of the lower classes, members of minority groups, transients, and residents of deteriorated urban areas; . . . criminal justice is founded on a stereotyped conception of the offender (e.g., drug user) as a pariah—a willful wrong doer who is morally bad and deserving of the community's condemnation and . . . confronted by public condemnation and the label of an evil [person], it may be difficult for an offender to maintain a favorable image of himself [or herself].[63]

In terms of drug use, a consistent pattern of events tends to take place resulting in a feedback cycle involving more deviations, more penalties, and still more deviations. Hostilities and resentment are built up, culminating in official reactions that label and stigmatize addicts, thereby justifying even greater penalties and restricting opportunities for the drug users to change their role. Often, drug offenders ultimately accept their deviant status and develop a career of systematic norm violations. It may be concluded from the labeling-criminalization process, therefore, that the treatment of drug law violators often serves as a self-fulfilling prophecy. It forecloses the offenders' noncriminal options and coerces them into a permanent state of drug use.

[I]t is common for addicts themselves to believe the conventional wisdom of "once an addict, always an addict," often expressed by them as having an "addictive personality," or being a "hope to die dope fiend." Such beliefs work to undermine users' decisions to stop and weaken their ability to resist relapse. . . . A second obstacle to addicts who are trying to end their drug abuse is the absence of any role model or subcultural folklore to give them insight into how they might implement their resolution. The reason for this lack of information about successful, self-initiated termination is that addicts who are able to maintain their abstinence without having utilized some form of treatment generally cease to associate with those who remain addicted. Consequently, successfully abstaining ex-addicts who remove themselves from the drug scene are believed to have failed in their resolve and, perhaps, are assumed to be readdicted in another city, imprisoned, or dead.[64]

BIOLOGICAL AND PSYCHOLOGICAL CHARACTERISTICS

Biological

"Biological theories are those that postulate innate, constitutional, physical mechanisms in specific individuals that impel them either to experiment with drugs, or to abuse them once they are exposed to them."[65] Research shows that certain individuals are predisposed toward drug and alcohol use because of their genetic makeup. Nondrinking sons, for example, have brain wave patterns similar to those of their alcoholic fathers.[66] Studies have showed that sons of alcoholics turned up with drinking problems four to five times as often as sons of nonalcoholics,[67] and it appears that genetic loading in combination with environmental and personality factors could make for a significantly higher level of drug abuse or alcoholism in certain individuals or groups in the population.[68] Another theory postulates metabolic imbalance as a possible cause of drug abuse—specifically, narcotic addiction.[69] While "no precise biological mechanism corresponding to metabolic imbalance has ever been located, the best that can be said about this theory is that the treatment program based on it, methadone maintenance, has helped a certain proportion of addicts."[70]

Psychological

Psychological theories associated with drug use and dependence may be categorized into two groups—those that emphasize the mechanism of reinforcement and those that stress personality differences between people who use and are dependent on drugs and those who abstain.[71]

In terms of the first approach, research shows that drugs have addicting reinforcement properties, independent of personality factors. There are two different approaches to understanding reinforcement theory—positive and negative. Positive reinforcement occurs when the individual receives a pleasurable sensation and, because of this, is motivated to repeat what caused it.[72] "The pleasure mechanism may . . . give rise to a strong fixation on repetitive behavior."[73] "The euphoria-seeking addict has sacrificed conventional activities and commitments for the hedonistic pursuit of pleasure; and to engage in this pursuit, a commitment to a deviant and criminal life-style is also necessary."[74] Negative reinforcement occurs when an individual does something to seek relief or to avoid pain, thereby being rewarded and, hence, motivated to repeat whatever it was that achieved relief or alleviated the pain. For example, "withdrawal symptoms as being due to the absence of opiates will generate a burning desire for the drug."[75] Addicts continue taking their drug of choice just to feel normal.[76]

Personality pathology, defect, or inadequacy is another theoretical approach. The inadequate personality approach points to problems of an emotional or psychic nature of certain individuals leading them to drug use. "They use drugs as an 'escape from reality,' as a means of avoiding life's problems and retreating into euphoric bliss and drugged out indifference."[77] This personality type lacks responsibility, independence, and the ability to defer pleasurable gratification for the sake of achieving long-range goals.[78] There is a tendency to use narcotics and hypnotics in order to manage such emotions as rage, shame, jealousy, and anxiety; to use stimulants to alleviate depression and weakness; to use psychedelics against boredom and disillusionment; and, to use alcohol against guilt, loneliness, and anxiety.[79]

This personality type also tends to have low self-esteem and feelings of self-derogation brought about by "peer rejection, parental neglect, high expectations for achievement, school failure, physical stigmata [rejection by the peer group], impaired sex-role identity, ego deficiencies, low coping abilities, and coping mechanisms that are socially devalued and/or are otherwise self-defeating."[80]

A focus on deviant or problem behavior reveals that those who use drugs, as compared to non-drug users, tend to be "more rebellious, independent, open to new experiences, willing to take a wide range of risks, accepting of deviant behavior and transgressions of moral and cultural norms, receptive to uncertainty, pleasure-seeking, hedonistic, peer-oriented, nonconformist, and unconventional. They also tend to be less religious, less attached to parents and family, less achievement-oriented, less cautious" and have a higher level of sexual activity.[81]

CONCLUSION

A number of theoretical approaches about drug use and dependence have been presented. What can be said about this information, beginning with the work of Dai[82] and Lindesmith,[83] is that it has contributed to nearly 50 years of debate and inquiry on the major views of the phenomenon—drug addiction as crime and drug addiction as disease—and to more recent descriptions of addicts and treatment programs.[84]

Many factors, either alone or in combination, influence or are associated with drug use and dependence.[85] These include (1) societal issues of normative structure, deviance definitions, and resources allocation; (2) sociological forces of the environment, values and morals, family, school, peers, and media and the labeling-criminalization process; and (3) biological/psychological personality characteristics. Figure 2.1 represents these factors as separate entities and in connection with each other.

NOTES

1. Ball, J., Nurco, D., Clayton, R., Lerner, M., Hagan, T., and Groves, G. (1995). Etiology, epidemiology and natural history of heroin addiction: A social science approach. In L. Harris (ed.), *Problems of Drug Dependence, 1994: Proceedings of the 56th Annual Meeting*. Vol. 1. Rockville, MD: NIDA, College on Problems of Drug Dependence, pp. 74–78.

2. Merton, R. (1969). Social structure and anomie. In D. Cressey and D. Ward (eds.), *Delinquency, Crime and Social Process*. New York: Harper and Row, pp. 254–284.

3. Merton, R. (1957). *Social Theory and Social Structure*. New York: Free Press.

4. Ibid., p. 188.

5. Cohen, A. (1965). The sociology of the deviant act: anomie theory and beyond. *American Sociological Review* 30: 5–14.

6. Cloward, R., and Ohlin, L. (1960). *Delinquency and Opportunity*. New York: Free Press; Palmer, S., and Linsky, A. (eds.) (1972). *Rebellion and Retreat: Readings in the Forms and Processes of Deviance*. Columbus, OH: Charles E. Merrill.

Figure 2.1
Factors Associated with Drug Use and Dependence

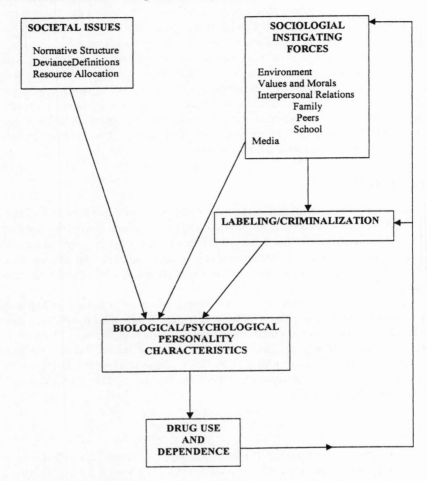

7. Lindesmith, A., and Gagnor, J. (1964). Anomie and drug addiction. In M. B. Clinard (ed.), *Anomie and Deviant Behavior: A Discussion and Critique*. New York: Free Press; Kandel, D. (1980). Drug and drinking behavior among youth. *Annual Review of Sociology* 6: 235–285; Goode, E. (1989). *Drugs in American Society*. 3rd ed. New York: McGraw-Hill, p. 64.

8. Reiss, A. (1965). *Schools in a Changing Society*. New York: Free Press, p. 57.

9. Goffman, E. (1963). *Stigma*. Englewood Cliffs, NJ: Prentice-Hall; Becker, H. (1963). *Outsiders: Studies in the Sociology of Deviance*. New York: Free Press.

10. Becker, p. 9.

11. Feldman, H., and Aldrich, M. (1990) The role of ethnography in substance abuse research and public policy: Historical precedent and future prospects. In Elizabeth Lambert

(Ed.), *The Collection and Interpretation of Data and Hidden Populations*, Monograph 98. Rockville, MD: NIDA, p. 19.

12. Shaw, C., and McKay, H. (1931). *Social Factors in Juvenile Delinquency: Report on the Causes of Crimes*. Washington, DC: National Commission on Law Observance and Enforcement, pp. 2–13; Shaw, C., and McKay, H. (1942). *Juvenile Delinquency in Urban Areas*. Chicago: University of Chicago Press; Lander, B. (1954). *Towards an Understanding of Juvenile Delinquency*. New York: Columbia University Press; Berkowitz, L. (1962). *Aggression: A Social Psychological Analysis*. New York: McGraw-Hill; Johnston, L., O'Malley, P., and Bachman, J. (1989). *Drug Use, Drinking and Smoking: National Survey Results from High School, College and Young Adult Population, 1975–1988*. DHHS Pub. No. (ADM) 89–1638. Washington, DC: U.S. Government Printing Office; Lorion, R., Bussell, D., and Goldberg, R. (1991). Identification of youth at high risk for alcohol or other drug problems. In E. Goplerud (Ed.), *Preventing Adolescent Drug Use: from Theory to Practice*. DHHS Pub. No. (ADM) 91–1725. Washington, DC: U.S. Government Printing Office, p. 71: Kvaraceus, W., and Miller, W. (1969). Norm-violating behavior and lower-class culture. In R. Caven (ed.), *Readings in Juvenile Delinquency*. Philadelphia: J. B. Lippincott.

13. Miller, W. (1958). Lower class culture as a generating milieu of gang delinquency, *Journal of Social Issues* 14, no. 3: 5–19.

14. Miller, W., Norm-violating behavior, pp. 5–19; Schrag, C. (1973). *Crime and Justice: American Style*. Rockville, MD: National Institute of Mental Health, pp. 71–80; Flay, B., and Petraitis, J. (1991). Methodological issues in drug use prevention and research. In C. Leukefeld and Bukoski, W. (Eds.), *Drug Abuse Prevention Intervention Research: Methodological Issues*. NIDA, DHHS Pub. No. (ADM) 91–1761. Washington, DC: U.S. Government Printing Office, p. 86.

15. Schrag; Cohen, A. (1955). *Delinquent Boys*. New York: Free Press.

16. Cloward and Ohlin.

17. Feldman, H., and Aldrich, M. (1990), The role of ethnography in substance abuse research and public policy: Historical precedent and future prospects. In E. Lambert (ed.), *The Collection and Interpretation of Data and Hidden Populations*. Monograph 98. Rockville, MD: NIDA, p. 20.

18. Schur, E. (1969). *Our Criminal Society*. Englewood Cliffs, NJ: Prentice-Hall, pp. 37–38.

19. Short, J., and Nye, I. (1957). Reported behavior as a criterion of deviant behavior. *Social Problems* (Fall): 207–213.

20. Clark, J., and Wenninger, E. (1970). Social class and delinquency. In M. Wolfgang, L. Savitz, and N. Johnston (eds.), *the Sociology of Crime and Delinquency*. New York: John Wiley and Sons; Scott, J., and Vaz, E. (1969). A perspective on middle-class delinquency. In Ruth Caven (ed.), *Readings in Juvenile Delinquency*. Philadelphia: J. B. Lippincott.

21. Kelley, H. (1952). Two functions of reference groups. In G. Swanson and T. Newcomb (eds.), *Readings in Social Psychology*. New York: Henry Holt; Wilson, W. (1987). *The Truly Disadvantaged: the Inner City, the Underclass and Public Policy*. Chicago: University of Chicago Press; Flay and Petraitis, Methodological issues, p. 86.

22. Merton, p. 282.

23. Berkowitz, p. 216.

24. Glynn, T., and Haenlein, M. (1988). Family theory and research on adolescent drug use: A review. *Journal of Chemical Dependency Treatment* 1, no. 2: 39–56.

25. Goodman, P. (1960). *Growing Up Absurd*. New York: Random House.

26. U.S. Office of Science and Technology (1973). *Youth: Transition to Adulthood. Report to the Panel on Youth of the President's Science Advisory Committee.* Chicago: University of Chicago Press.

27. Dinitz, S., Dynes, R., and Clark, A. (1975). *Deviance: Studies in Definition, Management and Treatment.* New York: Oxford University Press, p. 4.

28. Searcy, E., Harrell, A., and Grotberg, E. (1973). *Toward Interagency Coordination: an Overview of Federal Research and Development Activities Relating to Adolescence.* Washington, DC: Social Research Group, George Washington University, p. 27.

29. Whiting, J. (1971). An anthropological investigation of child-rearing practices and adult personality. In J. Segal (ed.), *the Mental Health of the Child.* Rockville, MD: National Institute of Mental Health; McCord, W., McCord, J., and Howard, A. (1961). Familial correlates of aggression in non-delinquent male children. *Journal of Abnormal Social Psychology* 62: 79–93; Elder, G. (1968). Adolescent socialization and development. In E. Borgotta and W. Lambert (eds.), *Handbook of Personality, Theory and Research.* Chicago: Rand McNally; Bandura, A., and Walters, R. (1959). *Adolescent Aggression: a Study of the Influences of Child Training Practices and Family Inter-relationships.* New York: Ronald Press; Goode, *Drugs in American Society,* pp. 62–67.

30. Robins, L., Davis, D., and Wish, E. (1977). Detecting predictors of rare events: Demographic, family and personal deviances as predictors of stages in progression toward narcotic addiction. In J. Strauss, H. Babigian, and M. Ross (eds.), *The Origins and Course of Psychopathology: Methods to Longitudinal Research.* New York: Plenum; Kandel, D. (1975). Adolescent marijuana use: Role of parents and peers. *Science* 181: 1067–1070; Kandel, D., Kessler, R., and Margulies, R. (1978). Antecedents of adolescent initiation into stages of drug use: A developmental analysis. *Journal of Youth and Adolescence* 7, no. 1: 13–40; Cooper, D., Olson, D., and Fournier, D. (1977). Adolescent drug use related to family support, self-esteem, and school behavior. *Center Quarterly Focus* (Spring): 121–134; Harbin, H., and Maziar, H. (1975). The families of drug abusers: A literature review. *Family Process* 14, no. 3: 411–431; Norem-Hebeisen, A., and Hedin, D. (1983). Influence on adolescent problem behavior: Causes, connections and contexts. In R. Isralowitz and M. Singer (eds.), *Adolescent Substance Abuse.* New York: Haworth; Needle, R. (1986). 35 Interpersonal influences in adolescent drug use: The role of older siblings, parents and peers. *The International Journal of the Addictions* 21, no. 7: 739–766; Simcha-Fagan, O., and Gersten, J. (1986). Early precursors and concurrent correlates of PG items of illicit drug use in adolescence. *Journal of Drug Issues* 60, no. 1: 7–28; Lorion et al., Identification of youth, pp. 75–76.

31. Copeland, J., and Howard, J. (1997). Substance abuse and juvenile crime. In Borowski, A., and O'Connor, I. (eds.), *Juvenile Crime, Justice and Corrections.* South Melbourne: Addison, Wesley, Longman, pp. 172–173.

32. Coombs, R., and Paulson, M. (1988). Contrasting family patterns of adolescent drug users and nonusers. *Journal of Chemical Dependency Treatment* 1, no. 2: 59–72.

33. Emmelkamp, P., and Heeres, H. (1988). Drug addiction and parental rearing style: A controlled study. *International Journal of the Addictions* 23, no. 2: 207–216.

34. Ball, J., Nurco, D., Clayton, R., Lerner, M., Hagan, T., and Groves, G. (1995). Etiology, epidemiology and natural history of heroin addiction: A social science approach. In L. Harris (ed.), *Problems of Drug Dependence, 1994: Proceedings of the 56th Annual Scientific Meeting.* Vol. 1. Rockville, MD: NIDA, College on Problems of Drug Dependence, pp. 74–78.

35. Yablonsky, L. (1969). The classification of gangs. In R. Caven (ed.), *Readings Injuvenile Delinquency*. Philadelphia: J. B. Lippincott; Goode, *Drugs in American Society*; Elliot, D., Huizinga, D., and Ageton, S. (1985). *Explaining Delinquency and Drug Use*. Beverly Hills, CA: Sage; Lubben, I., Kitano, J., and Harry, H. (1989). Differences in drinking behavior among three Asian American groups. *Journal of Studies on Alcohol* 50, no. 1: 15–23; Lubben, I., Kitano, J., and Harry, H. (1988). Heavy drinking among young adult Asian males. *International Social Work* 31, no. 3: 219–229; Austin, G., Prendergast, M., and Lee, H. (1989). Substance abuse among Asian American youth. *Prevention Research Update No. 5*. Portland, OR: Northwest Regional Education Laboratory (Winter): 1–13.

36. Cohen, A. (1955). *Delinquent Boys: The culture of the gang*. New York: Free Press.

37. Erickson, M., and Empey, L. (1969). Class position, peers and delinquency. In D. Cressey and D. Ward (eds.), *Delinquency, Crime and Social Process*. New York: Harper and Row, p. 417.

38. Kandel, D. (1980). Drug and drinking behavior among youth. *Annual Review of Sociology* 6: 235–285; Kandel, D. (1974). Inter- and intragenerational influences on adolescent marijuana use. *Journal of Social Issues* 30, no. 2: 107–135; Johnson, B. *Marijuana Users and Drug Subcultures*. New York: John Wiley and Sons; Goode, E. (1969). Multiple drug use among marijuana smokers. *Social Problems* 17 (Summer): 48–64; Goode, *Drugs in American Society*; Needle; Lorion, pp. 76–77.

39. Queipo, D., Alvarez, F., and Velasco, A. (1988). Drug consumption among university students in Spain. *British Journal of Addiction*, 83, no. 1: 91–98.

40. Kandel, D. (1980). Development states in adolescent drug involvement. In D. Lettieri, M. Sayers, and H. Pearson (eds.), *Theories on Drug Abuse: Selected Contemporary Perspectives*. Rockville, MD: NIDA, pp. 120–121.

41. Windle, M., Barnes, G., and Welte, J. (1989). Causal models of adolescent substance use: An examination of gender differences using distribution free estimators. *Journal of Personality and Social Psychology*, 56, no. 1: 132–142.

42. Ball et al., Etiology, pp. 74–78.

43. Copeland and Howard, Substance abuse, p. 172; Dielman, T., Butchart, A., Shope, J., and Miller, M. (1991). Environmental correlates of adolescent substance use and misuse: Implications for prevention programs. *International Journal of the Addictions* 25, nos. 7A, 8A: 855–880; Farrell, A. (1993). Risk factors for drug use in urban adolescents: A three-wave longitudinal study. *Journal of Drug Issues* 23, no. 3: 443–462; Hoffmann, J. (1993). Exploring the direct and indirect family effects on adolescent drug use. *Journal of Drug Issues* 23, no. 3: 535–557; Kandel, D., and Yamaguchi, K. (1985). Developmental patterns of the use of legal, illegal and medically prescribed psychotropic drugs from adolescence to young adulthood in *Etiology of Drug Abuse* (NIDA Research Monograph 56). Washington, DC: Department of Health and Human Services, pp. 193–235.

44. Cicourel, A., and Kitsuse, J. (1965). The social organization of high schools and deviant adolescent careers. in A. Reiss, Jr. (ed.), *Schools in a Changing Society*. New York: Free Press, p. 31.

45. Ahlgren, A., Norem-Hebeisen, A., Hochhauser, M., and Garvin, J. (1980). Antecedents of smoking among pre-adolescents. Unpublished paper; Smith, G., and Fogg, C. (1978). Psychological predictors of early use, late use, and non-use of marijuana among teenage students. In D. Kandel (ed.), *Longitudinal Research on Drug Use: Empirical Findings and Methodological Issues*. Washington, DC: Halstead-Wiley; Patan, S., Kessler, R., and Kandel, D. (1977). Depressive mood and adolescent illicit drug use: a longitudinal analysis. *Journal of Genetic Psychology* 131, no. 2: 267–289; Jessor, R., and Jessor, S.

(1977). *Problem Behavior and Psychological Development: A Longitudinal Study of Youth.* New York: Academic Press; Bachman, J., O'Malley, P., and Johnston, D. (1978). *Adolescence to Adulthood: Change and Stability in Lives of Young Men.* Ann Arbor, MI: Survey Research Center; Millman, D., and Wen-Huey, S. (1973). Patterns of illicit drug use among secondary school students. *Journal of Pediatrics* 83, no. 2: 314–320; Smith, G. (1975). Teenage drug use: A search for cause and consequences. In D. Lettieri (ed.), *Predicting Adolescent Drug Use: a Review of Issues, Methods and Correlates.* DHEW Pub. No. (ADM) 276–299. Washington, DC: National Institute on Drug Abuse; Newcomb, M., and Bentler, P. (1989). Substance use and abuse among children and teenagers. *American Psychologist* 44, no. 2: 242–248; Hawkins, J., Lishner, D., Catalano, R., and Howard, M. (1985). Childhood predictors of adolescent substance abuse: Toward an empirically grounded theory. *Journal of Children in Contemporary Society* 18, no. 1–2: 11–48.

46. Schooler, C., and Flora, J. (1996). Pervasive media violence. *Annual Review of Public Health* 17: 275.

47. Klapper, J. (1960). *The Effects of Mass Communication.* New York: Free Press.

48. Banay, R. (1955). *Hearings Before the United States Senate Subcommittee to Investigate Juvenile Delinquency.* U.S. Senate Committee on the Judiciary, Television Programs and Juvenile Delinquency, 84th Congress, First Sessions, pp. 81–83. Washington, DC: U.S. Government Printing Office.

49. Behavior USGSACoTaS. (1972). *Television and Growing Up: the Impact of Televised Violence: Report of the Surgeon General, Us Public Health Service.* Washington, DC: U.S. Government Printing Office.

50. Pearl, D., Bouthilet, L., and Lazar, J. (1982). *Television and Behavior: Ten Years of Scientific Progress and Implications for the Eighties.* Washington, DC: U.S. Government Printing Office.

51. Fine, G., Mortimer, J., and Roberts, D. (1990). Leisure, work, and the mass media. In S. Feldman and G. Elliot (eds.), *At the Threshold: The Developing Adolescent.* Cambridge: Harvard University Press, pp. 225–252.

52. Christenson, P., and Roberts, D. (1990). *Popular Music in Early Adolescence.* Washington, DC: Carnegie Council on Adolescent Development; Klein, J., Brown, J., Childers, K., Oliveri, J., Porter, C., and Dykers, C. (1993). Adolescents' risky behavior and mass media use. *Pediatrics* 92: 24–31.

53. Gerbner, G., and Gross, L. (1976). Living with television: The violence profile. *Journal of Communication* 27: 171–80.

54. Cohen, B. (1963). *The Press and Foreign Policy.* Princeton: Princeton University Press.

55. Heath, L., Bresolin, L., and Rinaldi, R. (1989). Effects of media violence on children. *Archives of General Psychiatry* 43: 376–379.

56. Singer, J., Singer, D., and Rapaczynski, W. (1984). Family patterns as predictors of children's beliefs and aggression. *Journal of Communication* 34: 73–89; Singer, J., and Singer, D. (1981). *Television, Imagination, and Aggression: a Study of Preschoolers.* Hilldale, NJ: Erlbaum.

57. Berkowitz, p. 244.

58. Ibid., p. 255.

59. Atkin, C. (1990). Effects of televised alcohol messages on teenage drinking patterns. *Journal of Adolescent Health Care* 11, no. 1: 10–24.

60. Hughes, E. (1984). The study of occupations. *The Sociological Eye: Selected Papers.* New Brunswick, NJ: Transaction Books, pp. 283–297.

61. Becker, H. (1963). *Outsiders: Studies in the Sociology of Deviance*. Glencoe, IL: Free Press.

62. Becker, H. (1953). Becoming a marijuana user. *American Journal of Sociology* 59: 235–242; Feldman, H., and Aldrich, M. (1990). The role of ethnography in substance abuse research and public policy: Historical precedent and future prospects. In E. Lambert (ed.), *The Collection and Interpretation of Data for Hidden Populations*. Monograph Series 98. Rockville, MD: NIDA, U.S. Department of Health and Human Services, p. 19.

63. Schrag, pp. 89–92.

64. Biernacki, P. (1990). Recovery from opiate addiction without treatment: A summary. In Elizabeth Lambert (ed.), *The Collection and Interpretation of Data from Hidden Populations*. NIDA Research Monograph 98. Rockville, MD: NIDA, U.S. Department of Health and Human Services, pp. 113–119.

65. Goode, *Drugs in American Society*, p. 55.

66. Kolata, G. (1987). Alcoholism: Genetic links grow clearer. *New York Times*, November 10, pp. C1, C2; Kumpfer, K. (1988). Prevention of substance abuse: A critical review of risk factors and prevention strategies. In D. Shaffer and I. Phillips (eds.), *Project Prevention*. Washington, DC: American Academy of Child and Adolescent Psychiatry.

67. Goodwin, D. (1971). Is alcoholism hereditary? *Archives of General Psychiatry* 25: 545–549; Goodwin, D. (1979). Alcoholism and heredity: A review and hypothesis. *Archives of General Psychiatry* 36: 57–61; Goodwin, D. (1984). Studies of familial alcoholism: A review. *Journal of Chemical Psychiatry* 45, no. 2: 14–17.

68. Schucket, M. (1980). A theory of alcohol and drug abuse: A genetic approach. In Lettieri, Sawyers, and Pearson, *Theories on Drug Abuse*; McCord, J. (1988). Alcoholism: Toward understanding genetic and social factors. *Psychiatry* 51, no. 2: 131–141.

69. Dole, V., and Nyswander, M. (1965). A medical treatment for diacetylmorphine (heroin) addiction. *Journal of the American Medical Association* 193 (August): 646–650; Dole, V., and Nyswander, M. (1980). Methadone maintenance: A theoretical perspective. In Lettieri, Sawyers, and Pearson, *Theories on Drug Abuse*; Dole, V. (1980). Addictive behavior. *Scientific American* 243 (December): 138–154.

70. Goode, *Drugs in American Society*, p. 57.

71. Ibid.

72. Ibid., pp. 57–58.

73. Bejerot, N. (1980). Addiction to pleasure: A biological and social-psychological theory of addiction. In Lettieri, Sawyers, and Pearson, *Theories on Drug Abuse*, p. 253.

74. Goode, *Drugs in American Society*, p. 60.

75. Sutter, A. (1966). The world of the righteous dope fiend. Issues in *Criminology* 2 (Fall): 195.

76. Goode, *Drugs in American Society*, pp. 58–59.

77. Ibid., p. 60.

78. Ausubel, D. (1980). An interactionist approach to narcotic addiction. In Lettieri, Sawyers, and Pearson, *Theories on Drug Abuse*, pp. 4–5.

79. Wurmser, L. (1980). Drug use as a protective system. In Lettieri, Sawyers, and Pearson, *Theories on Drug Abuse*.

80. Kaplan, H. (1980). Self-esteem and self-derogation theory of drug abuse. In Lettieri, Sawyers, and Pearson, *Theories on Drug Abuse*, p. 129.

81. Goode, *Drugs in American Society*, p. 62.

82. Dai, B. (1937). *Opium Addiction in Chicago*. Shanghai: Commercial Press (Reprint, Montclair, NJ: Patterson Smith, 1970).

83. Lindesmith, A. (1947). *Opiate Addiction*. Bloomington, IN: Principia Press, 2nd ed., *Addiction and Opiates*. Chicago: Aldine, 1968.

84. Hanson, B., Besschner, G., Walters, J., and Bovelle, E. (1985). *Life with Heroin: Voices from the Inner City*. Lexington, MA: Lexington Books; Biernacki, P. (1986). *Pathways from Heroin Addiction: Recovery Without Treatment*. Philadelphia: Temple University Press.

85. Conroy, R. (1988). The many facets of adolescent drinking. *Bulletin of the Menninger Clinic* 152, no. 3: 229–245; Smart, R. (1986). Solvent use in North America: Aspects of epidemiology, prevention and treatment. *Journal of Psychoactive Drugs* 18, no. 2: 87–96; Flay and Petraitis, Methodological issues, pp. 81–109; Lorion et al., Identification of youth, pp. 53–89.

Chapter 3

Heroin: The "King" of Illegal Drugs

HISTORICAL PERSPECTIVE

If one substance were to be labeled the "king" of illegal drugs, most people would say it is heroin. Since the turn of the century, when it was created, heroin has virtually defined the drug problem.[1]

Disapproval of any level of use is higher for heroin than it is for any other drug; opposition to legalization is higher for heroin than it is for any other drug; and heroin addicts are the most stigmatized of all drug users. Heroin is the epitome of the illicit street drug. Its association in the public mind with street crime . . . in spite of strong competition from crack, is stronger than for any other drug. The stereotype of the "junkie" is that he or she is by nature a lowlife, an outcast, a dweller in the underworld, an unsavory, untrustworthy character to be avoided at almost any cost.[2]

Heroin is chemically derived from morphine, which in turn comes from the opium poppy, grown primarily in the Golden Triangle located in parts of Thailand, Laos, and Burma (now Myanmar), the Golden Crescent, which creates a border between Afghanistan, Pakistan and Iran, the Middle East, most notably, Lebanon, and Latin American countries including Colombia and Mexico. Opium is the product of the poppy plant, *papaver somniferum*, an annual plant growing three to four feet high, with a long-stemmed large (four to five inches in diameter) flower that is either purple, red, pink, white, or scarlet, depending on the species. The plant grows in mountainous areas, although not at very high altitudes. Once the flower opens, the bulb is slashed or punctured with a three-pronged knife, and the flowing juice, once dried by the wind, is collected. This dried substance is then boiled until it becomes a mass of raw opium called "black." Black is then refined to a morphine base, which is later transformed into heroin. Each successive step requires more sophisticated laboratory techniques, although the first steps can be made directly in the fields, where a good part of the opium is consumed, often eaten by natives in the areas where the plant is grown.

The word "opium" is derived from the Greek word for juice, and literary critics have suggested that the sailors who accompanied Ulysses in the *Odyssey*, whom Homer described in the ninth century B.C. as eating lotus, were actually consuming opium; the Country of the Lotophagi would, according to this version, be located in the Far East. "The first historical reference to opium is on a wall plaque from 2,000 B.C. found in Kurgia, Turkey. The four edges of the plaque are decorated with opium poppy pods. The first written description of the use of opium is on a papyrus called the *ibis papyrus*, dated between 1550 and 1600 B.C. The papyrus points out some of the salient therapeutic uses of opium, even in those days, for pain and for constipation."[3] Opium and the opium poppy had been known to the Chinese well before the year 1000, when it was primarily used by a select, elite group. Over the years, the Chinese developed the habit of smoking tobacco and eating opium. Eventually, these two pleasures became one (i.e., in the form of smoking), and opium became the substance of choice.[4] Arab merchants trading in the Silk Route knew it as "amdak" and they introduced it to the West as a medicinal plant in the seventh and eighth centuries A.D. The Chinese name for the substance was "Chandu," or "Yen" (this is the origin of the English word "yearn"), and it became "Akbari" when introduced to India. Opium preparations were part of the armamentarium of every self-respecting Arab doctor in a period when Arab medicine was probably the best in the world. Opium over time has been used against malaria, colitis, and pain.[5]

By 1729, the use of opium in China was so prevalent that a law was introduced mandating that opium shop owners were to be strangled. Once opium for nonmedical purposes was outlawed, it was necessary for the drug to be smuggled in from India, where poppy plantations were abundant.[6] The economic stakes were high for those involved; smugglers included British adventurers and members of the British East India Company. It has been noted that "the British had very little success with introducing alcohol either in India or the Far East. A certain percentage of the Asian population have enzyme systems that cause them to have severe side effects from the ingestion of alcohol. Thus, until recently, alcohol was not popular in [that region of the world]. The British decided to go into the opium business, and they were joined by all the other Western powers. They grew opium in India and exported it to China."[7] When an effort was made in 1839 to suppress the smuggling of opium into China, relations among nations and peoples became strained, resulting in the Opium War of 1839, which lasted for about two years. "As victors, the British were given the island of Hong Kong, broad trading rights, and $6 million to reimburse the merchants whose opium had been destroyed."[8] Not until 1906, through the British Parliament, was legislative action taken to stem the opium trade, but by that time problem behavior related to opium addiction was no secret, especially among those who provided the substance. "There were at the end of the Second World War, hundreds of thousands of opiate dependent individuals in the People's Republic of

China. These by and large disappeared from view, at least until very recently, when there has been a resurgence in opiate use."[9]

In 1806, a young German scientist by the name of Frederich Sertürner published a report on his isolation of the primary active ingredient in opium—an ingredient ten times more potent than opium itself. Sertürner named it "morphium" after Morpheus, the god of dreams. Two major developments during the nineteenth century promoted the widespread use of morphine. First, in 1853 the hypodermic syringe was perfected by Dr. Alexander Wood, making it possible to introduce morphine directly into the bloodstream or body tissue rather than the slower process of eating opium or morphine and waiting for it to be absorbed through the gastrointestinal tract. The second factor was the use of morphine as a pain relief agent for casualties of the American Civil War (1861–1865), the Prussian-Austrian War (1866), and the Franco-Prussian War (1870). The percentage of returning veterans from those wars addicted to morphine was high enough that the illness was later called "soldier's disease" or the "army disease."[10]

In 1874, a chemical bonding process for morphine was discovered that produced heroin—a substance about three times as potent as morphine. Initially marketed by Bayer Laboratories of Germany in 1898 as a nonaddictive substitute for codeine, derived from opium, it took nearly a decade of research before it was found that heroin was the most addictive of the opiates, able to affect brain functioning faster than anything yet known.

Despite a growing problem of opiate dependence arising from unrestrained distribution of opium derivatives within the medical system in the United States, it was the street use of the opiates and cocaine that generated public and professional interest in their habit-forming properties. After the U.S. Civil War, it appears that a host of conditions arose that were to lead to various city, state, and federal legislation attempts to control the spread of drug use. Among these factors were increased Chinese immigration on the West Coast that was linked to smoking opium, the possession of opium pipes, and the maintenance of opium dens; the addicted Civil War soldiers; and the widespread use of patent medicines for the relief of aches, pains, and anxiety that contained alcohol and/or opiates such as opium or morphine and that could be legally purchased at the a store or through mail order firms like Sears Roebuck.[11]

Although estimates varied, it was generally believed that the total number of addicts never exceeded a quarter of a million, divided evenly between medical and street dependence. Increased awareness, brought about by crusades waged among law enforcement officials against the street use of opiates and cocaine, aroused public anxiety about a narcotics problem of major proportions. The movement for national alcohol prohibition further sensitized the public to a need for national drug prohibitions; the culmination was the passage of the Harrison Narcotics Act of 1914 in the United States.[12]

This act outlawed non-medical use of opiates, and Supreme Court decisions during the next seven years further narrowed even the medical uses of opium products. With the Harrison

Act, people who had become dependent on opiates had to seek alternative sources for drugs containing opiates. This elimination of the medical supply of opiates and the criminalization of opiate use shifted narcotic addiction from the medical arena to the legal arena. At the same time, this law precipitated the need for treatments to assist those who were addicted to opiates but could no longer obtain them from their physicians.[13]

Following the Second World War, "the enactment of anti-opium laws in many parts of Asia in which opium use was traditional—India, Hong Kong, Thailand, Laos, Iran—effectively suppressed the availability of opium at the cost of stimulating the creation of domestic heroin industries and substantial increases in heroin use. The same tradition had occurred in the United States following Congress's ban on opium imports in 1909."[14] It has been noted that at the turn of the century:

despite the virtual absence of any controls on availability, the proportion of Americans addicted to opiates was only two to three times greater than today. . . . The typical addict was not a young black ghetto resident but a middle-class white Southern women or a West Coast Chinese immigrant. The violence, death, disease, and crime that we today associate with drug use barely existed, and many medical authorities regarded opiate addiction as far less destructive than alcoholism (some doctors even prescribed the former as treatment for the latter). Many opiate addicts, perhaps most, managed to lead relatively normal lives and kept their addictions secret even from close friends and relatives. That they were able to do so was largely a function of the legal status of their drug use.[15]

With a ban on opiates, new forces entered the market, namely, the illegal organizations interested in making a quick profit. Those organizations succeeded in popularizing the opiates in the United States and Europe much faster than the British had succeeded in China. Until the mid-1960s, laboratory facilities to transform morphine base into heroin were available only in Europe and the United States. This meant that most of the product had to be transported to be refined, and the refining process put a great deal of money into Western hands. In the mid-1960s two apparently unrelated episodes changed the situation. On one hand, under American pressure, the Turkish government agreed to close most of the illegal fields in that country, reserving a small portion of the product for legal medicinal purposes. On the other hand, Hong Kong-based drug entrepreneurs succeeded in establishing a series of laboratories in the field along the Mekong River. They started refining the product locally.

[It is rumored that] those organizations foresaw the massive American intervention in the Vietnam War and readied themselves to profit from the American soldiers coming to the area. Others claim that the Vietcong foresaw American intervention and assisted the Chinese in establishing the laboratories, so that heroin could be easily available in order to support the war effort. . . . Also, it is claimed that the political changes undergone by Vietnam at the time were related, at least partially, to the war for the domination of the heroin market. . . . President Diem, his brother Nhu who ran the opium traffic at that time, and Madame Nhu were deposed and assassinated. They were succeeded in the government by General Ky who was also deeply involved in the opium trade business. . . . At that time, the Laotian and

Burmese armies were involved; the United States Central Intelligence Agency [is alleged to have] organized the traffic through a number of small airlines such as Air Laos Commercial (also known as "Air Opium"); and Kuomintang soldiers (Chinese nationalists) escorted the caravans transporting the raw material to Saigon, Bangkok and other places. The alleged reason for the CIA supporting the traffic was related to the American need to provide economic support for allied countries to prevent them from turning communist.[16]

Up to the early part of this decade, evidence revealed no significant rise in opiate and heroin addiction despite the general impression to the contrary.[17] For example, about 1 percent of all Americans have tried heroin at least once in their lives, but among those who have used any illegal drug, fewer than 3 percent have tried or used heroin.[18] Among all episodes of illegal drug use only 1 percent involve heroin.[19] Presently, however, surveys reveal that illegal drug use is on the rise, especially among young people. According to the European Monitoring Center on Drugs and Drug Addiction, the most alarming trend is heroin use. "It has long been the biggest source of Europe's drug-related crime and medical problems, including AIDS and hepatitis from shared needles. Now its availability and popularity are growing."[20] In the early 1990s the European addict population, estimated at between 500,000 and one million, seemed to stabilize. Now, in most places, heroin has gotten cheaper, purer, and easier to find than before. For example, the price has dropped to a level that is cheap enough to smoke or snort the substance instead of injecting it, making it attractive for those who want to experiment. One reason for this is geopolitics. Since the end of the Cold War, drugs have been financing some of the religious and ethnic conflicts. According to Interpol:

[T]he warlords have become the drug lords . . . the collapse of the Soviet Empire opened up new supply routes and spawned smuggling rings from Burma to Estonia. The opening of borders in the European Union afforded unprecedented access to a vast untapped market. Aggressive criminal gangs in Africa and South America have been quick to seize the initiative, too. Capitalizing on skills in dealing marijuana or cocaine, they have expanded their product lines to include heroin . . . with a significant amount being South America heroin which was virtually unknown five years ago. In 1994 it accounted for 32 percent of the heroin seized in America; last year (1995) it was up to a "staggering 62 percent."[21]

While South American producers and marketers have made major gains dealing with heroin, the first name in the product line is China white, which comes from Southeast Asia's Golden Triangle. In China white, Asian heroin syndicates believe they have found their answer to cocaine: a drug (i.e., heroin) they can sell to the middle class. Designated officially as No. 4 heroin, China white is the purest heroin ever marketed; it is also plentiful and relatively cheap. In New York, where it is sold in glassine envelopes under names such as Dynamite, Ferrari, and White Death, China white accounts for more than 70 percent of the heroin sold. Middle-class heroin users are increasingly attracted to China white. Its greater purity means that users need less of it to get high. In addition, they can snort or smoke the powder, a relatively clean and discreet way of taking the drug that avoids the risk of catching AIDS from infected needles or suffering a fatal overdose from shooting up.

This new-style heroin abuser can become an addict as readily as someone using a needle. But smoking or sniffing is less likely to be instantly fatal: usually a user will nod out before absorbing lethal quantities of heroin. [An official of the New York office of the Drug Enforcement Administration—DEA] says that many cocaine and crack addicts have taken to using heroin as well. Heroin's mellow euphoria is a counterpoint to what he calls the "hyperkinetic effects" of cocaine and crack. . . . According to the National Institute of Drug Abuse, the number of intravenous heroin users has remained constant from 1982 [to 1991]: 492,000 addicts nationwide, with half of them located in New York. The numbers of heroin-related cases in U.S. hospital emergency rooms—one of the standard barometers of the drug's inroads—also have changed little from 1988 to 1991. [Yet, it was predicted then by U.S. drug experts and law enforcement officials that there were ominous signs of a heroin comeback with improved purity at much lower cost.][22]

TRENDS

Have the predictions of increased heroin use and the problems associated with its abuse proved correct? The answer is yes, for the most part, based on epidemiological trends reported by the U.S. National Institute on Drug Abuse. The following are highlights of the heroin situation in the United States up to 1996 as reported by the National Institute of Drug Abuse (NIDA):[23]

In several areas throughout that country, heroin mortality increased and heroin was found to be the most frequent illicit, nonalcoholic drug mentioned in emergency room reports. In [many cities], heroin is the top-ranking primary drug of abuse (excluding alcohol only and alcohol in combination) among treatment admissions.

Use Patterns: While the "old time" users continue to inject heroin and strive for a heroin high, more recently initiated users are more likely to snort or smoke heroin and use it as a means to cope with the negative side effects of crack cocaine use. Among the latter, an increasing number . . . are shifting to injecting heroin as they no longer get the desired effect from snorting or smoking it. . . . Users also reported that unlike several years ago, dealers now say that the product is good enough to inhale. . . . New users, while they begin drug use by inhaling, are reported to move quickly to injecting the drug . . . some snorters are former IDUs [injecting drug users] who have switched to smoking rock and snorting heroin, either because injecting is difficult or because they fear AIDS. A small but increasing number of these people also reported smoking heroin. . . . Since snorting is familiar and doesn't carry the stigma of injecting drug use, the present population of cocaine users becomes a new potential cache of heroin users. . . . Street sources indicated younger people are snorting heroin mixed with cocaine, and older heroin addicts are continuing to inject. . . . There are reports from the African-American community of young users "shaking up heroin in Visine bottles," then spraying it into the nose. . . . Hispanic immigrants . . . prefer the injection route. . . . Hispanics are . . . "shabanging," which is picking up the cooked heroin with a syringe and squirting it up their nose. A variation of this practice is called "usando aqua de chango" (using the monkey water), and an eye or nose dropper is used instead of a syringe. . . . As is the case with cocaine, mode of heroin administration is often correlated with demographic characteristics. For example, in Newark, the proportion of snorters is higher among female admissions than males and among African-Americans than among whites or Hispanics; and, in New York City, intranasal users are more likely than injectors to be female, to be younger by 2 or 3 years, and to be Hispanic or African-American. . . . In some areas, such as New York City, addicts snort heroin in the street in open view; some, however, prefer shooting galleries because they fear being robbed by crack addicts.

Multisubstance Use and Shifting Use Patterns: Street sources indicate that more users are mixing heroin and cocaine and smoking it. . . . Snorting of heroin has spread to cocaine abusers. Use of cocaine appears to be a significant risk factor for initiating heroin use . . . one researcher was told, "I use dope to come down from crack so I can go back up" . . . a small but increasing number of these people also report smoking heroin, either alone, as "chasing the dragon," or in combination with crack cocaine, as a "speedball" . . . there is a new practice called criss-crossing that involves placing a straw in each nostril sniffing separate lines of heroin and cocaine, and crossing straws when halfway through.

Demographics:

(Age) The latest data measuring incidence of heroin consequences are now confirming previous anecdotal reports of the drug's abuse spreading to newer and younger populations . . . the 26–34 age group still accounts for the highest rates of mention per 100,000 population in every city . . . there is evidence of an aging cohort of injectors growing . . . focus group and outreach workers reported that heroin is attracting new users who are primarily white, male, and in their teens. . . . Mortality figures in some cities confirm anecdotal reports of three emerging types of heroin users: a small, but growing number of younger users relatively new to the heroin scene; crack users who are starting to combine their crack with heroin; and a larger population of aging addicts who are switching to intranasal use (and sometimes smoking) . . . new users [e.g., in Philadelphia] are likely to be white, male, and between the ages of 14 and 18 or 19.

(Gender) Males predominate in heroin mortality figures . . . males also outnumber females as a percentage of heroin emergency department mentions . . . among primary heroin treatment admissions, males account for the majority [of clients].

(Race/Ethnicity) Decedents were predominately white in most areas reporting heroin mortality. . . . Emergency department admissions show mixed racial demographics . . . · and among heroin treatment admissions the results are mixed depending on the racial composition of the city (e.g., in New York, Hispanics are the largest group; in Los Angeles, the largest groups are whites and Hispanics; in Miami the largest group is whites; and in Detroit, blacks are the largest group of heroin addicts seeking treatment).

Law Enforcement Data (Availability): Lower priced, higher quality heroin remains widely available [in many locations] with supplies coming from Colombia, Southeast Asia and Southwest Asia. In New York City, $5-bag brand names include "rush," "do or die," "expressway delivery," "powder," and "checkmate." . . . Lower quality heroin from Mexico still predominates in most western areas [of the United States].

(Price and Purity): Referring to the $5 bags, a drug user commented that "the dope is better and just as much as you get in a dime bag." . . . One observer noted, "China white is in town, but it's very expensive." . . . In many locations, heroin purity is increasing and the price is declining. . . . Heroin contaminants are reported . . . scopolamine (sometimes known as "polo")—combined with dextromethorphan, quinine, or in some cities with heroin or even cocaine—has been sold as heroin . . . the term "polo" refers to the entire drug combination . . . such combinations have been dubbed "homicide" and "super buick." . . . "Wicked," the brand of heroin linked with the outbreak of overdose episodes in Chicago, is purportedly cut with strychnine, according to unconfirmed reports. . . . Other Chicago brands associated with those episodes include "rawhide," "raw fusion," "tootsie roll," "big foot," "sledge hammer," and "graveyard."

THE HEROIN ADDICT: PERSONALITY CHARACTERISTCS

There are many theories about why people use and abuse heroin and other harmful substances, including those discussed in Chapter 2. In terms of inadequate personality, addicts have been found to lack responsibility, independence, and the ability to defer gratification in order to achieve long-range goals.[24] They are unable to face realities of life, confront their problems, or meet the demands of society[25] and have difficulty controlling emotions such as rage, shame, jealousy, and anxiety.[26] They tend to have low self-esteem,[27] with feelings of "peer rejection, parental neglect, unrealistic expectations for achievement, school failure, physical stigmatism (e.g., devalued group memberships), impaired sex role identity, ego deficiencies, low coping abilities, and (generally) coping mechanisms that are socially devalued and/or are otherwise self-defeating."[28]

Research on deviance and problem behavior has found that those who use and abuse drugs such as heroin tend to be more rebellious and are willing to take a wide range of risks that often involve socially unacceptable behavior transgressing moral and cultural norms.[29] Such persons are receptive to uncertainty and are inclined to be pleasure-seeking and hedonistic, peer-oriented, and nonconformist, as well as unconventional.[30] "Users also tend to be less religious, less attached to parents and family, less achievement-oriented, and less cautious. This personality manifests itself in a wide range of behavior, much of it not only unconventional, but problematic for the individual and for mainstream society."[31] In this context, one factor is most common—heroin users and addicts are closely associated with a life of crime. These people "tend to be recruited from social circles in which deviance, delinquency and crime are more acceptable and more common than average."[32] Heroin users have extremely high rates of criminal behavior, especially with respect to money-making crimes. Inciardi[33] described the level of heroin-related crime as "astronomical." Discounting drug offenses, there were more than 230 criminal offenses per year per user—from procuring and prostitution to armed robbery and assault. These drug users are more involved with crime than others who use illegal substances. What emerges from research is that the use of, or addiction to, narcotic drugs seems to intensify a tendency to be involved in criminal activity[34] and consequently to increase an addict's relation to the criminal justice system. Prison for such offenders is generally considered to be the option of last choice. It represents the inability or unwillingness of the family, service agencies, and/or the justice system (e.g., police and courts) to continue the support of the heroin addict in the community because of severe functional limitations and behavioral problems.

Generally speaking, heroin addicts have many characteristics in common. Using a status model perspective, however, the question arises whether certain psychological factors differ based on the nature of treatment services received (e.g., heroin addicts imprisoned because of drug offenses and those self-referred to a community outpatient treatment program). The following factors were used to determine the differences: (1) attitude toward drug taking; (2) interpersonal relationships, including those with parents, siblings, and peers; (3) self-concept in terms of the addicts' perception about their own abilities, success or failure in life, and happiness or unhappiness; (4) personal values on perspectives of human nature, the world, honesty, and dedication to society; (5) risk-taking tendency; (6) motivation; (7) rebelliousness against rules and regulations, social institutions, and authorities; and (8) pleasure-seeking. Findings show only two psychological characteristics significantly different among the prison and community-based addicts: attitudes toward using drugs and attitudes toward pleasure. For both characteristics, community-based heroin addicts reported a greater inclination toward illegal drug use and self-gratification. Additional results regarding the psychological factors of heroin addicts show that liberal attitudes toward illegal drug use were more common among those who had a lower self-concept, and were more likely to take risks, more rebellious, and more pleasure seeking. Those with positive interpersonal relations were likely to have a positive self-concept and to be less likely to be risk takers and more motivated. Positive self-concept was related to positive personal values and motivation. Positive personal values were linked to motivation and a lesser degree of rebelliousness. Risk taking was found to be correlated with those who were more rebellious and pleasure seeking. Those with a greater degree of motivation were less rebellious. Rebelliousness was linked to pleasure seeking.[35]

The status model of drug use among heroin addicts shows that the psychological characteristics of prisoners are no more (and in some cases even more positive) than those in a community-based treatment program. This finding is somewhat surprising, considering the negative status associated with those assigned to prison, a placement of last resort, but understandable considering the controlling effect prison may have on the attitudes and behavior of addicts. Imprisoned addicts, more than those in a community-based treatment program, tend to attitudinally reject illegal drug use and pleasure-seeking experiences (e.g., altered state of consciousness).[36]

CROSS-CULTURAL PERSPECTIVE OF HEROIN ADDICTS

The use of illegal substances such as heroin may be the result of a number of factors, including those of a personal, social, and/or cultural nature. From a cross-cultural perspective, one question that arises is to what extent addicts from different countries have common attitudes toward the use and abuse of heroin.

To assess such a question, an adequate selection of countries must be made, and considerations, including those based on economic, political, cultural, and other relevant factors, need to be taken into account. While drug use has seldom been systematically studied in a cross-national or cross-cultural manner, it should be recognized that considerable exploratory work is necessary, and there can be no guarantee that the most rigorous research will provide definitive results. With this in mind, research was conducted in Singapore and Israel to test whether location is related to the attitudes, norms, and behavior of addicts toward drug use. The study included 100 heroin addicts in Singapore and an equal number who claimed never to have used illegal substances.[37] These two groups were compared to 109 heroin addicts and 76 non-drug users in Israel.[38]

The ethnic background of the heroin and non-drug users in Singapore was 76 percent Chinese, 22 percent Malay and 2 percent other. In Israel, 95 percent of the participants were Sephardim (Jews of Middle Eastern origin), and 5 percent other. Personal factors controlled were age (18–30); sex (male); education (high school education or less); and socioeconomic status (low income). All subject data were collected with a pretested questionnaire of a self-report, anonymous nature and used to test the concept of status model and heroin addiction described earlier. The questionnaire included factors of attitude toward drug taking; interpersonal relationships; self-concept; personal values; risk-taking tendency; motivation; rebelliousness, and pleasure seeking. Results regarding the psychological characteristics of the heroin addicts revealed that those from Singapore, compared to their Israeli counterparts, have a more positive profile in terms of interpersonal relations, self-concept, personal values, and motivation. The Singapore heroin addicts, however, tended to be more pleasure seeking, risk taking, and inclined to continue using illegal drugs. The only characteristic shared among the addicts from both countries was rebelliousness.

Among the non-drug users, significant psychological differences were found to exist on seven of the eight scales used. In every situation, except the tendency toward risk taking, which showed no significant difference between subjects of both countries, the participants from Singapore tended to have a more positive psychological profile based on the factors studied. Specifically, they reported a more law-abiding attitude toward drug taking, as well as better interpersonal relations, self-concept, personal values orientation, and motivation. Also, they reported being less pleasure seeking and rebellious.

Clearly, a societal and cultural explanation of psychological character formation is best supported by the findings of the non-drug users. The Singapore participants report a strong, positive profile, much more so than their Israeli counterparts. While the findings of this study are exploratory in nature, which limits generalization, a number of interesting response patterns emerged that are worthy of further investigation. First, Singapore is a small but dynamic society dominated by a rather homogeneous Chinese culture and heritage that strongly endorse positive personal and familial values.[39] It is not surprising, therefore, that the study participants from that island/nation, regardless of their drug use status, report more positive attitudes than those from Israel, which is much more culturally diverse. How these results would compare to a different socioeconomic group of Israeli people such as those with a Northern and Eastern European background, is open to further query.

Another finding that should be investigated is the considerable degree of response similarity among heroin addicts and non-drug users in Israel to the questions used. It is possible that the personality characteristics use in this study do not differentiate heroin addicts and non-drug users in Israel with the same ethnic and socioeconomic background. The results of this binational comparison show that heroin addicts have few psychological characteristics in common, and the differences tend to be influenced by the prevailing social and cultural norms of the society in which they reside.[40]

HEROIN ADDICTION: CASE EXAMPLES

The Case of C

C was in his early 20s when he came for treatment. He was the second of eight children from a relatively stable family with a good economic situation. The family income came from work as a greengrocer with a stand at an open market. All of the family worked at the stand, and C loved the job. He talked often about the excitement of the place, the shouting, the pushing up of sales, the competition with other grocers for a client, and the haggling over a price. That was his life, what he really liked to do.

C studied eight years at a elementary school and started high school, but the attraction of the market was stronger, so he quit his studies and dedicated all of his time to the stand. According to him, at age 14 his earnings were more than those of an average worker. With lots of money from his work, C bought clothes for himself, his sisters, of whom he was very fond, and his friends, with a considerable amount left over. This inevitably attracted the attention of addicts and pushers, who were common around the market. In this environment, C began smoking hashish and attending parties with people older than himself. At the parties he felt the need to show that he was on an equal basis with others there and that he could do exactly what older people were doing. The problem was that what the older people were doing was taking drugs, so C started using heroin at the age of 16.

In the beginning it was easy, and it was fun. C had no money problems, so he could afford relatively large amounts of heroin. He had found that the drug had an excellent, relaxing effect on him—he felt calm, he was able to interact with other people better, and he was able to sit down for hours on end, something he had not been able to do before. Also, he could enjoy sex in a relaxed and calm way. Through the personal strengths and abilities he found through heroin, C was better liked by other people, and as a result of the acceptance he was very happy.

This initial period in the life of an addict is known as the "honeymoon," which has a time span dependent on all kinds of circumstances, mostly economic ones. In this period, addicts rarely get into trouble except if they try to buy or sell heroin to an undercover police agent. For C the "honeymoon" did not last very long. In spite of his good salary, he found himself without sufficient resources to buy the increasing amount of heroin he needed.

At age 17, he committed his first crime when he attacked an elderly lady on the street. He snatched her gold chain and medallion, which he immediately traded for heroin. He remembered very well that he consumed all of the heroin that same day, so the next day he had to go out and rob again. Soon he had to go out every night to steal in order to maintain his habit; and by the age 18 he had become a well-known housebreaker. He would rob at least two apartments a week as well as continue to work at the market for the money and because he did not want his family to suspect he was involved in drugs and criminal activity.

Continuously in a drugged state, C's production had diminished to the extent that his father, still not suspecting anything wrong, complained about his "laziness," calling him a "bum" and asking him not to continue to work at the stand. His dismissal came after an episode in which a substantial amount of money disappeared from the stand's cash drawer. C claimed that he had nothing to do with the episode and that he would not steal from his own family; nevertheless, knowing what heroin can do to the judgment of people under its influence, the possibility that he took the money cannot be ruled out. After being fired from the stand, C lost the only link he still had with a "normal" life and became more involved with drugs and the underworld.

C was first caught by the police at age 19 and served a short sentence at a special prison for young adults and first-time offenders. While in prison he continued to use huge amounts of drugs, and since he was unable to pay, he found his way to heavy debts and even bigger problems. Once released, he went back to work in order to make a living and to pay back his debts because heroin debts are as sacred as gambling debts, and not paying them has very serious consequences for the debtor. Creditors cannot forgive a debt, not necessarily because of the money involved but because all of their control over the people they are involved with resides in their ability to recover their money, no matter what the circumstances or the amount. If they failed to do so, they would be out of business in no time.

C succeeded in staying out of jail for six months until he was caught again, this time for housebreaking and possession of drugs. He received a one-year sentence from a rather benevolent judge. In prison he kept the same lifestyle as the first time, and when released, he was deeper in debt than before, so the same pattern followed, and he found himself in jail for the third time, this time for three years. At this crisis stage, his drug involvement became so well known that help was finally offered to him.

When first examined for treatment, he had already undergone detoxification, and from his history and the examination it was clear that C suffered from minimal brain dysfunction (MBD). MBD is a well-recognized but badly defined condition appearing mostly in children. No clear organic lesion can be identified, but the disease is characterized by a pattern of hyperactivity, lack of concentration, lack of patience, and school performance generally below what would be expected from the person's I.Q. The poor school performance of the patient is generally attributable to a lack of concentration and hyperactivity. Although the condition appears first in childhood, it may extend well into adulthood and sometimes accompanies the patient throughout life. There is an accepted treatment for the condition, the so-called paradoxical treatment. In this treatment, a drug that is generally hyperactivating, such as amphetamines (speeds) or Methylphenidate (also an amphetamine-like substance), is administered to the patient. Instead of enhancing the hyperexcitation, the drug reduces the state of hyperexcitation and produces a return to a normal or near normal pattern of behavior.

C was informed of the diagnosis and treatment plan. Unfortunately, he refused to accept the medication and insisted that he was not "sick." He knew he had a "drug problem" but insisted he could overcome it with some help—"conversation" was all he needed. Nevertheless, C was referred to a therapeutic community, where he stayed for well over a year. There he used heroin occasionally but denied it even when traces of the substance were found in his urine.

Other than that, he did reasonably well under treatment—he showed an adequate understanding of his problem and stopped his illegal activities. He was progressing "satisfactorily" in treatment according to the therapist; however, when seen interacting in group therapy, there were serious doubts about his progress. Just before his departure from treatment to a rehabilitation center, a last attempt was made to convince C to accept the "paradoxical treatment" for his MBD, without success.

The condition of C at the rehabilitation center was followed through reports from the therapist who stayed in touch with him. He continued doing apparently "well" until he was released six months after his admission. According to the information provided by other patients who worked at the same market as C, it was not surprising to learn that he had gone back to drugs a few months after treatment, that he was back in jail and was looking bad as a result of the symptoms associated with withdrawal. C was offered, once again, the needed "paradoxical treatment"; however, his mumbled and somewhat incoherent response was something to the effect that he was "perfectly able to solve his own problems with just a little help"—"conversations" were again all he needed. That was the last time C was seen. Shortly after receiving a 5-year sentence for burglary and drug possession, C committed suicide. He was 25 years old.

The case of C is very sad because almost everything related to his debilitating condition could have been avoided if the necessary intervention measures had been taken at the correct time. C was not been born and raised in a remote village, nor did his parents lack the money for treatment. C had undergone all the routine health checkups as a child; however, it was the failure on the part of school personnel not to have noticed that C suffered from MBD. His parents may have lacked the knowledge to understand that he had a problem, but the health professionals who took care of him over time should have detected the condition. When he dropped out of school, the officer in charge of finding out the reason for such action should have considered the possibility of a dysfunction of some sort. MBD is common enough to be on the mind of every educator or health authority so that it can be detected and treated. In the case of C, the condition went undetected for years. Nobody did anything, nobody warned the parents, nobody offered treatment, nobody worried, nobody cared. As a result, C became a delinquent and a drug addict and died long before his time. But not everything must be attributed to educators, physicians, and parents. Although all these persons may be held responsible for not detecting the condition, the final result, the suicide, was due to something else—the "world of heroin" and a false sense of pride felt by C.

When C came for treatment it was recognized that he was deeply involved in the underworld and drugs just by looking at his forearms. They were covered with signs of slashing. Slashing is a more telltale sign than injection marks. Addicts usually slash for different reasons; for example, it is considered a means of protest against some "arbitrary" measure taken by the authorities; and it is done in prison to receive medical attention, providing the addict with an opportunity to steal medicine. Most often, slashing is a means of breaking a very painful withdrawal syndrome. The slashing produces a release of endorphins that calm the patient. In the first few minutes after the slashing, the process is much less painful for the addict than one would suppose. On one occasion, people who had slashed less than 10 minutes before they were brought to the clinic had to be sutured. They could have been sutured without anesthetics, and they would not have felt the suture needle entering their skin. The pain began to be felt by them 10 to 15 minutes after slashing—up till then the patient felt relaxed and almost exultant, having broken, at least temporarily, the abstinence syndrome. Slashing means that the patient has no drugs available and is ready to do just about anything to procure heroin. A person who has slashed has to be watched because it may be a precursor to suicide or an attack on somebody. C had learned the trick during his first prison term and had used it profusely. His left forearm was full of scars, and his right forearm also showed marks.

In the case of C, his false sense of pride forbade him to accept the condition of "sick" and in need of treatment because any condition attributable to something related to the brain is seen as "psychiatric." The person automatically becomes a "psycho," thus descending several steps in the underworld's social status. The fact that MBD is really a neurological condition rather than a psychiatric one is irrelevant; the underworld does not accept such distinctions. C committed suicide because he found himself unable to continue his life pattern of crime and drug dependence; he did not know how to get out of the situation he had got himself in. He was having difficulty getting drugs and found himself in a condition of almost permanent withdrawal suffering, which is a very painful condition. He could have asked for help, and help would have been made available for him immediately, but he had already failed once and probably did not have the necessary strength left to swallow his pride and come back for treatment. He had to find another way out, and he chose the one truly definitive way out.

The Case of E

E was a small female, aged 25, when she was admitted to the psychiatric hospital for intense depression that accompanied a serious attempt at suicide. Her history was rather typical of many young women from the streets of the red-light district.

She was the third of four daughters in her family; her father was religious and chronically unemployed; her mother was a small, shy figure who obeyed her husband as though he were God himself. She worked outside the home to support the family. E started school at a normal age and was screened at age 7 by a school psychologist and a school nurse without evidence of any special problems. At age 9, E was raped by her father—apparently a family tradition. Her two older sisters had also been raped by the father at age 9 as well and were sent to work as prostitutes at age 12 in order to support the family. This story was confirmed by one of E's sisters, who was a heroin addict.

E reluctantly started working and making money as a prostitute. She would frequently run away and hide from her father; however, he usually found her after a few days and would beat her until she agreed to continue the work. At 14, E started using hashish, reportedly to avoid vomiting while performing oral sex with some of her clients. She was introduced to heroin at 15 by one of her father's friends who received her favors for free. The man, thankful for her attention, gave her heroin as a reward. By 16, E was heavily addicted and started injecting from time to time, although most of her consumption was by inhaling. At that time she was caught by police and taken to an institution for juvenile offenders. In the institution she learned how to inject in hidden places, such as in her groin, to avoid detection of the needle marks. Also, while there she learned new sexual tricks and made new connections. During her time in treatment she reported how she and one other inmate would run away at night to work for one hour or two in the streets in order to make money to buy heroin and hashish, which they brought back to the institution and shared with their friends. They would also commit small robberies when possible.

E was 18 when her father died. In spite of the abuse she has received from him, she felt remorse and a sense of guilt, believing that his death was the result of her misbehavior and God's way to punish her for her sins. She decided to quit heroin use, so she sought help at a mental hospital, where she received ambulatory treatment. With the help of her sister, who would keep her company and comfort her, she succeeded with detoxification by locking herself up in her room.

She dealt with the intense suffering of the cold turkey by slashing her wrists and her abdomen when she was no longer able to bear the pain. After 10 days, the pain of withdrawal finally started receding, and E believed she was drug-free, so she left her room. She had lost about 10 percent of body weight in the process and felt very weak but very happy. One week after leaving her room, E ventured out of the house to visit some friends and give them the good news that she was clean. When meeting them she was offered heroin, which she tried to refuse, but one of her former sources took hold of her and forcibly injected her with the substance, compelling her to take up prostitution again. The process was repeated several times, and after a week or so she was addicted again.

E continued working as a prostitute to support her pimp, who was providing her with the drug. Asked why she had not tried to run away at that stage instead of wasting all the suffering of the cold turkey, E explained that it was impossible to run away. She mentioned the case of a girl she had known who had tried to run away. Her pimp looked all over for her, and when he found her he ordered some of his people to kill her in the most brutal way so that she would be an example to other girls. Her corpse was found a few days later by the police. She had been slashed and had bled to death, and the corpse was rat-bitten. No other girl dared to escape after that incident.

E was arrested again at the age of 20 and was prosecuted for possession of heroin for personal consumption. She was sentenced to six months of actual prison with a one-year conditional sentence. While she served her term her pimp was also arrested and charged with several offenses that carried a heavy sentence—in a way E was free. She decided to run away from her familiar environment, heroin, and her past. Unfortunately, she had not taken into consideration her conditional sentence. She was detained at the airport and confined to her house. Once there the usual pattern of behavior returned and E started working the streets and using heroin once more. She became so depressed that she tried to commit suicide. She swallowed all the pills she could get hold of, more than 100, all kinds.

The suicide attempt was "serious" because E did not know that the amount of pills she had taken would not kill her. Many people have the tendency to swallow a large number of pills, believing that such a large quantity will be fatal. That is not necessarily so. Death depends on the kind of pill more than on the number, but the number of pills ingested gives us a fair indication of the seriousness of the attempt. Usually, a suicide attempt made with a large number of nonfatal pills is considered to be more serious than an attempt made with a smaller number of fatal pills.

E's attempt failed, and she was taken to a general hospital, where her condition was evaluated by a psychiatrist as being "depressed" and "drug-addicted." Instead of admitting her to a psychiatric hospital, the psychiatrist prescribed antidepressant pills and treatment on an ambulatory basis. E did not accept the recommendation, and the moment she left the general hospital, she went back to heroin and prostitution.

The episode leading to her admission to the psychiatric hospital for treatment started when one of her friends, a young girl of 18, died of an overdose without medical attention after having been brutalized, raped, and overinjected by her pimp and some friends. The reason for the punishment was that she had committed the "crime" of keeping some of her earnings for herself instead of turning them all over to her pimp, who in turn would provide her with a small amount of pocket money and heroin. E was so shocked over the incident that she became acutely depressed and again tried to commit suicide—this time by slashing her wrists. She was found unconscious in a public toilet and carried to a general hospital, from which she was transferred to a psychiatric hospital for treatment.

By the time she received the treatment that was needed, E had overcome most of the withdrawal syndrome but was very depressed. She remained at the hospital for more than six months and received the usual antidepressive treatment and psychotherapy. She was anxious to cooperate and do well; however, she left the hospital against medical advice, wishing once again, to move away from her familiar environment to try to start a new life in a place where nobody knew her and where there were no drugs. After two months of hiding in another city where she had been working as a waitress in a small restaurant, E had been found by her pimp and his two friends. She was forced to return to her previous life and habits.

The case of E provides insight into the world of heroin and demonstrates the influence of the environment on the development and maintenance of drug addiction. The girl's father was a deviant but by no means a very strange or unusual one. A history of incest and rape is a frequent factor in the life of an addict, especially among women but also among men. Incest is much more frequent than thought, and it is not necessarily related to rape unless it involves a child. Incest is seldom reported, and too often it is not only accepted but even sought by the child, indicating pathology in the family.

In the world of heroin use, a women is not a person—she is an object with a very well defined role as a provider. Prostitution is an accepted and almost normal situation for a female heroin addict. Of course, the form of prostitution may change with the social conditions. A girl from a lower-class background will most probably walk the streets, while a girl with higher status may find easier ways of prostituting herself. In the end, both are prostitutes. An ex-addict from a relatively well-to-do family who had never worked the streets in her life classified herself as an ex-prostitute when she considered her past experiences from her own perspective. Though she did not receive money for her sexual favors, she always obtained heroin through sexual intercourse with men who either had money to buy the drug or had access to it through other ways. Her experience was just another form of prostitution.

The role of provider attributed to, or imposed on, female heroin addicts makes them very valuable. Their defection from such a role is considered a big economic loss, and a pimp will go to great lengths to secure the return of one of his girls, because a street girl can make several hundred dollars a night with her work. The pimp needs that money to subsist and to provide heroin for both of them. Running away from that situation is very difficult, as in the case of E. The underworld has connections everywhere. A network of informants causes almost everybody in the underworld to be under more or less permanent surveillance even when out of the direct reach of close associates. Once a runaway is detected bringing her back is of considerable importance since she has hurt the pride and social status of her "owner." To teach a lesson to other possible runaways, the runaway may be brutalized or killed directly by the "owner" or by a proxy. In cases where being brutalized is the response, especially when the women is still young and productive, the woman's face will be preserved as much as possible, or only light damage will be caused, because a beautiful prostitute makes more money. When killing is the option, as was the case with the friends of E, it is usually done in a very ugly manner to stress the undesirability of running away.

Providing heroin to a street girl is only a way of dominating her, not of making her happy or unhappy. A heroin-addicted street girl is dependent forever on a constant supply of the drug, and she will not try to run away from her pimp because otherwise she would be cut off from her source. Even if she runs away and finds a new source of heroin, the new provider will likely put her to work for him in exchange for the heroin. In that way, the situation of the girl remains basically unchanged, and she will continue on the streets as long as she is able to make money. Once the heroin-addicted woman ages and is no longer able to earn money as a prostitute, it is likely that she will not live long because of health problems. Such women be found in all kinds of institutions, like hospitals and jails, although sometimes they succeed in becoming valuable after their active phase has passed as trainers of younger prostitutes. Old ex-prostitutes very often turn to alcohol, which is much cheaper than heroin, but they soon succumb to the combination of alcoholism and malnourishment and usually develop some serious disease that leads them to the tomb or to a mental institution. That will probably be future of E, too.

The case of E is a typical one in the sense of the depression that accompanies heroin or cocaine addiction. Some statistics place the incidence of "mental disorders" as high as 70 percent among addicts. This figure includes psychosis, depression, personality disorders, and other problems. The incidence of "depression" alone can be as high as 40 percent or more. Since little is known about the origin of depression, and less is known about the factors leading to addiction, it would be bold to establish any kind of causal relationship, but the relationship, causal or not, definitely exists. That relationship may be responsible for the high incidence of suicide attempts among addicts. As mentioned earlier, these attempts may be clear-cut or disguised in all sorts of ways, but they cause the death of a large number of addicts. If all the estimates are put together, a rough total of 20 percent to 25 percent of the addicts commit suicide. In a report issued by the U.S. Substance Abuse Treatment and Mental Health Services Administration "suicide attempt or gesture" was the most commonly reported motive for taking a substance and constituted 37 percent of all drug-related episodes in 1996.[41]

NOTES

1. Kaplan, J. (1983). *The Hardest Drug: Heroin and Public Policy*. Chicago: University of Chicago Press; Goode, E. (1989). *Drugs in American Society*. New York: McGraw-Hill.

2. Goode, p. 226.

3. Harris, L. (1993). Opiates: A history of opiates and their use in treatment. In C. Hartel (ed.), *Biomedical Approaches in Illicit Drug Demand Reduction*. Rockville, MD: NIDA, p. 85.

4. Ray, O., and Ksir, C. (1990). *Drugs, Society and Human Behavior*. St. Louis, MO: Times Mirror/Mosby College, p. 274.

5. Telias, D. (1991). *The World of "H."* Tel-Aviv: Freund Publishing House.

6. Scott, J. (1969). *The White Poppy: A History of Opium*. New York: Funk and Wagnalls.

7. Harris, p. 89.

8. Ray and Ksir, p. 275.

9. Harris, p. 90.

10. Lindesmith, A. (1965). *The Addict and the Law*. Bloomington: Indiana University Press; Ray and Ksir, *Drugs, Society,*, p. 278; Weisberger, B. (1993). The Chinese must go. *American Heritage* (March): 24–26.

11. Musto, D. (1973). *The American Disease: Origins of Narcotic Control*. New Haven, CT: Yale University Press; Nadelmann, E. (1993). Should we legalize drugs? History answers. *American Heritage* (March): 41–48.

12. Ray and Ksir, p. 280.

13. McCann, M., Rawson, R., Obert, J., and Hasson, A. (1994). *Treatment of Opiate Addiction with Methadone*. Rockville, MD: U.S. Department of Health and Human Services, p. 2.

14. Nadelmann, p. 45.

15. Ibid.

16. Telias, p. 6.

17. Johnston L., O'Malley, P., and Bachman, J. (1987). *National Trends in Drug Use and Related Factors among American High School Students and Young Adults 1975–*. Rockville, MD: NIDA; Martz, L. (1990). A dirty drug secret. *Newsweek*, February 19, p. 44.

18. National Institue of Drug Abuse (NIDA). (1986). *Highlights of the 1985 National Household Survey on Drug Abuse*. Rockville, MD: NIDA.

19. Goode, p. 228.

20. Dickey, C., and Underhill, W. (1996). The drug threat. *Newsweek*, October 14, pp. 41–47.

21. Ibid., p. 43.

22. Liu, M. (1991). The curse of china white. *Newsweek*, October 14, pp. 10–16.

23. NIDA. (1996). *Epidemiologic Trends in Drug Abuse*. Vol. 1: *Highlights and Executive Summary*. Rockville, MD: U.S. Department of Health and Human Services.

24. Ausubel, D. (1980). An interactionist approach to narcotic addiction. In D. Lettieri, M. Sayers, and H. Pearson (eds.), *Theories on Drug Abuse: Selected Contemporary Perspectives*. Rockville, MD: NIDA, pp. 4–7.

25. Scher, J. (1970). Patterns and profiles of addiction and drug abuse. In J. McGrath and F. Scarpitti (eds.), *Youth and Drugs*. Glenview, IL: Scott, Foresman, pp. 25–29.

26. Wurmser, L. (1980). "Drug use as a protective system." In Lettieri, Sayers, and Pearson, *Theories on Drug Abuse*, pp. 71–74.

27. Jurich, A., and Polson, C. (1984). Reasons for drug use: Comparison of drug users and abusers." *Psychological Reports* 55: 371–378; Smart, R., and Whitehead, P. (1974). The uses of an epidemiology of drug use: The Canadian scene. *The International Journal of the Addictions* 9: 373–388.

28. Kaplan, H. (1980). "Self-esteem and self-derogation theory of drug abuse." In Lettieri, Sayers, and Pearson, *Theories on Drug Abuse*, pp. 128–131.

29. Lukoff, I. (1974). Issues in the evaluation of heroin treatment. In E. Josephson and E. Carroll (eds.), *Drug Use: Epidemiological and Sociological Approaches*. New York: Wiley, pp. 129–157; Jessor, R., and Jessor, S. (1977). *Problem Behavior and Psychosocial Development: a Longitudinal Study of Youth*. New York: Academic Press; Kandel, D. (1973). "Adolescent marijuana use: Role of parents and peers." *Science* 181 (September 14): 1067–1070.

30. Jessor and Jessor, *Problem Behavior*; Jessor, R., and Jessor, S. (1980), A social-psychological framework for studying drug use. In Lettieri, Sayers, and Pearson, *Theories on Drug Abuse*, pp. 102–109.

31. Goode, p. 62.

32. Goode, p. 235.

33. Inciardi, J. (1979). Heroin use and street crime. *Crime and Delinquency* 25 (July): 335–346; Inciardi, J. (1986). *The War on Drugs: Heroin, Cocaine, Crime and Public Policy.* Palo Alto, CA: Mayfield, pp. 122–132.

34. Inciardi, *The War*, pp. 130–140; Goode, *Drugs*, p. 236.

35. Isralowitz, R., Telias, D., and Zighelbaum, Y. (1992). Heroin addiction in Israel: A comparison of addicts in prison, community-based facilities, and non-drug users based on selected psychological factors. *International Journal of Offender Therapy and Comparative Criminology* 36, no. 1: 70.

36. Ibid.

37. Ong, T. (1989). *Drug Abuse in Singapore: A Psychological Perspective.* Singapore: Hillview.

38. Ong, T. H., and Isralowitz, R. (1996). *Substance Use in Singapore: Illegal Drugs, Inhalants and Alcohol.* Singapore: Toppan, pp. 135–144.

39. Ibid., p. 143.

40. Ibid., p. 144.

41. Substance Abuse and Mental Health Services Administration (1997). Drug-Related Emergency Room Cases Decline Nationally, SAMHSA Press Office, December 30.

Chapter 4

Alcohol and the Alcoholic

HISTORICAL PERSPECTIVE

While many substances have been used to experience special physical sensations, alcohol has remained the most important over time. Alcohol is a drug in precisely the same sense that heroin, cocaine, and LSD are—they are all psychoactive. Alcohol is "addictive," and in this sense definitions regarding dependence and abuse are parallel to what is presented in Chapter 1 under definitions for "substances." It generates severe withdrawal symptoms when the heavy, long-term drinker discontinues its use. It has been noted that because withdrawal from alcohol can be a physically and psychologically difficult process, including symptoms such as depression, blackouts, and liver disease, some individuals who are dependent on the substance may continue to use alcohol despite adverse consequences to avoid the symptoms of withdrawal. According to the *Diagnostic and Statistical Manual of Mental Disorders* (DSM—4th Edition), "a substantial minority of individuals who have Alcohol Dependence never experience clinically relevant levels of Alcohol Withdrawal, and only about 5% of individuals with Alcohol Dependence ever experience severe complications of withdrawal (e.g., delirium and grand mal seizures)."[1]

When a person abuses alcohol to the point that school and job performance suffers, child care or household responsibilities are ignored, and there is a range of social and interpersonal problems including violent arguments with spouse, child abuse, and other problem behavior, and "problems are accompanied by evidence of tolerance, withdrawal, or compulsive behavior related to alcohol use, a diagnosis of Alcohol Dependence, rather than Alcohol Abuse, should be considered."[2] Alcohol abuse and dependence are by far the most common form of drug addiction. In the United States, it is estimated that there are 10 million alcoholics and only half a million heroin addicts.[3]

Although it is not known exactly when alcohol and its effects on human behavior were discovered, paleontologists say that the four basic ingredients needed to produce the substance (i.e., sugar, water, yeast, and heat) have existed as long as 200 million years and in almost all geographic locations and cultures.

[There is] ample testimony from Ancient Egyptians, Hebrews, Greeks, and Romans that intoxicating beverages, both wines and stronger drinks, were well known within their cultures. Alcohol may be the most popular drink in recorded history. We know humans have been drinking alcoholic beverages since 6400 B.C., when beer and berry wine were discovered. Grape wines date from 300 to 400 B.C. . . . The drinking custom is probably even older than that. Some experts believe that mead, an alcoholic beverage made of honey, was used about 8000 B.C. . . . The destruction of individuals and families by excessive, irresponsible drinking has been recorded as well. One of the oldest temperance [accounts] was written in Egypt, about 3,000 years ago under the title of the "Wisdom of Ani" stating "Take not upon thyself to drink a jug of beer. Thou speakest and an unintelligible utterance issueth from thy mouth. If thou fallest down and thy limbs break there is none to hold out a hand to thee. Thy companions in drink stand up and say 'away with this sot,' and thou art like a child." Reference to alcoholism is in the Bible (Chapter 1 of the First Book of Samuel). As told by Keller, Hannah was childless and extremely unhappy on account of it. At the annual family pilgrimage to the shrine in Shiloh she could not partake of the festal meal. She went off by herself and stood, leaning against the wall of the shrine, praying to God to grant her a son. She prayed silently, only her lips moving but she made no sound. Eli, the high priest, noticed her odd behavior and mistook this gentlewomen for a hallucinating drunkard and advising that an alcoholic must give up drink altogether.[4] Leaders throughout history have encouraged moderation. King Solomon warned the ancient Hebrews to beware of alcohol. Plato and other Greek philosophers urged their followers likewise. In ancient times, an intoxicated person was often shunned and condemned. . . . In China, wine drinking prohibitions were enacted and repealed 40 times between 1100 B.C. and A.D. 1400.[5]

Early use of alcohol seems to have been worldwide; for example, beer was drunk by the American Indians encountered by Columbus.[6] Wine drinking was common in medieval Britain, and consumption was high. When William of Orange became king of England in 1688, he encouraged the production of gin by issuing charters to divert the surplus of English grain for its production. In 1690, a further step to ensure the sale of English grain was taken when import of foreign spirits was prohibited. In Queen Anne's time, the monopoly of the Worshipful Company of Distillers was canceled, leading to unlimited gin production, mostly of poor quality, which was sold in the streets and hawked from door to door at one penny per pint.[7] Ale has been drunk in England since Celtic times, and hopped beer since the fifteenth century.[8] The tragedy of drunkenness was summed up in the eighteenth century, when it was said that "some of the most dreadful mischiefs that afflict mankind proceed from wine. It is the cause of disease, quarrels, sedition, idleness, aversion to labor, and every species of domestic disorder."[9]

In the "new continent," what American colonists considered normal drinking would be defined as deviant and intemperate from a contemporary viewpoint. "The colonists" views toward alcoholics were reflective of their basic philosophic assumptions regarding free will and moral depravity of human beings, and of their class bias."[10] Levine[11] notes that between 1785 and 1835 considerable concern about drinking by the poor was being expressed among an economic and social elite.

In the United States in 1784 Benjamin Rush, a physician and signer of the Declaration of Independence, described in his work "An Inquiry into the Effects of Ardent Spirits upon the Human Body and Mind" that drunkenness was a disease resembling certain hereditary, family and contagious diseases.[12] In nineteenth-century America, a temperance movement that "demonized" alcohol became an important social force and a rallying point for the expanding middle class; thus, the liquor problem became a focus of attention for a broader sector of American society[13] that would bring social, political, and religious activism together, culminating in Prohibition. In the United States, an amendment to the Constitution in 1919 made it illegal to manufacture or sell any alcoholic beverage. This amendment remained in effect until 1933 and had a significant impact on the nation's social patterns, economy, and underground life during those years and after.[14]

The end of Prohibition, it has been suggested, was the result not so much of an overwhelming American popular desire for legitimate sources of alcohol but of corporate interests that saw the restoration of liquor taxes as a means of lowering personal and business taxes.[15] Moreover, at a time when social and economic pressures and protests due to the Great Depression were building, popular disregard of Prohibition was also viewed as another aspect of disregard for law and order.[16] Once Prohibition was repealed, the windfall from taxes on alcohol was used to fund depression relief projects.[17]

No record of alcohol sales was kept in the United States from 1920 to 1933; nevertheless, there is a general perception that alcohol consumption rose during this period and that Prohibition was a failure. Contrary to this belief, death by cirrhosis of the liver, which is very closely correlated with alcohol consumption decreased during Prohibition and increased once alcohol use was legal again.[18] The number of people arrested and jailed on charges of public drunkenness and the number of automobile fatalities, another factor strongly related to the consumption of alcohol, declined as well.[19] Exaggeration, myths, and the media probably account more for the misunderstanding of Prohibition's effect on people's drinking behavior than any other factors. "In general, most Americans did not drink during [this period], and those who did drank significantly less, and less often, than they did before or after."[20]

Over time, the detrimental results of alcohol use have been subject to a macabre array of remedies to address the problem. For example, Pliny the Elder in his Historia Naturalis (xxxii, 49), written in the first century, suggested putting a roach or worm or other disgusting creature (e.g., screech owl's eggs) into the drink of a drunkard to stop excessive use of wine. In 1601, a book was published in England recommending the use of a tonic wine in which eels or green frogs had been suffocated to wean the uncontrolled drinker. The Chinese used both human cerumen (i.e., earwax) and the head of a rat ashed in the first moon as medicaments for the treatment of alcoholism. In more recent times, the Ruthenians—a group of Ukrainians living in Ruthenia and eastern Czechoslovakia—believed that the problem of excessive alcohol use could be dealt with by pouring the drunkard's own urine back into his mouth, while the Magyars believed the problem could be cured by secretly mixing sparrow's dung into the drunkard's brandy. Also, the Ruthenians believed that alcoholism could be cured by placing a piece of pork secretly into a Jew's bed and keeping it there for nine days, then pulverizing it and feeding it secretly to the drunkard. This was done in the belief that the drunkard will abhor alcoholic drink as a Jew abhors pork. Throughout the nineteenth century, the notion of secretly mixing "special" substances into the drink or even coffee of alcoholics was a popular way to try to cure the problem. In places like Brazil such a practice continues. It has been reported that Dr. Benjamin Rush once tempted a patient who was habitually fond of ardent spirits to drink some rum in which he had put a few grains of tartar emetic. The tartar sickened the patient and caused him to vomit, believing that he had been poisoned. Dr. Rush was gratified by observing that the patient could not bear the sight or smell of alcohol for two years afterward.

One hundred and fifty years later, Doctor Walter Voegtlin, who had not read Rush but had read Pavlov, was to develop the same idea into a systematic method using emetine to induce vomiting in association with alcohol. This treatment helped several thousand alcoholic patients to become total abstainers. Doctor Rush himself, never having heard of Pavlov, credited the idea to no less an authority than Moses when, he writes, Moses compelled the children of Israel to drink the solution of the golden calf (which they had idolized) in water. This solution, if made as it probably was, by means of what is called hepar sulphuris, was extremely bitter, and nauseous, and could never be recollected afterwards, without bringing into equal detestation, the sin which subjected them to the necessity of drinking it.[21]

TRENDS

There can be little doubt that the magnitude of alcohol use and problems associated with its use have been overshadowed in recent years by the preoccupation with the widespread use of drugs such as heroin, cocaine, and crack, as well as the threat of AIDS, but "[t]ake the deaths from every other abused drug . . . add them together, and they still don't equal the deaths or the cost to society of alcohol alone."[22] In the United States alone, alcoholism claims tens of thousands of lives each year, ruins untold numbers of families, and costs from $85.8 billion[23] to $117[24] billion a year in everything from medical bills to lost workdays. The primary chronic health hazard associated with alcohol use is cirrhosis of the liver. Cirrhosis is among the leading causes of mortality in the United States and is attributed to alcohol use.[25]

Alcohol use has been targeted as the cause for nearly half of all driving fatalities in the United States[26] and is the major factor in adult drownings.[27] It has been seriously implicated in millions of injuries and thousands of deaths resulting from industrial accidents and a substantial proportion of general (noncommercial) aviation crashes and boating accidents. The vast majority of all fire fatalities and fire burns involve alcohol use at the time of the accident—cigarette smoking is a major cause of fires, and a direct association exists between drinking and smoking in the general population. Alcohol has been found to be involved in up to 70 percent of all deaths and 63 percent of all injuries from falls. Suicide is a major cause of death in the United States, and about 30 percent of those who commit suicide are alcoholics.[28] Alcoholics are far more likely than nonalcoholics to attempt and commit suicide while drinking, and alcohol's mood-changing properties have been seen as a possible link to suicidal actions. Child abuse, neglect, molestation, and marital violence are prevalent types of aggression in the family, and alcohol use is a precipitating factor of these problems as well.[29]

A Department of Justice survey estimates that nearly a third of the nation's 523,000 state prison inmates drank heavily before committing rape, burglaries, and assaults. As much as 45 percent of the country's more than 250,000 homeless are alcoholics.[30] In the 1989 Bureau of Justice Statistics survey of inmates in local jails throughout the United States, offenders charged with, or convicted of, driving while intoxicated were more than one in every 11 inmates. Among convicted inmates, 86 percent of those serving a sentence for driving while intoxicated (DWI) had a prior sentence to probation, jail, or prison for a DWI offense or other offense. Almost a third of the DWI inmates had served three or more previous sentences in jail or prison. Regarding those who are arrested for driving while impaired, persons in jail for DWI are more likely to be the serious offenders in terms of the nature of criminal activity.[31]

The use of alcohol in the United States rose steadily from the end of Prohibition to 1978. For the last ten years or so, however, there has been a downward trend—a behavior pattern that appears in consonance with the use of most psychoactive substances, with cocaine as the one major exception. Other factors characterizing the downward trend of alcohol use during the past decade include a decline in sales, decreased self-reported alcohol consumption for all ages, and fewer young people ever drinking.[32] Alcohol-related traffic fatalities dropped from 25,165 in 1982 to 17,699 in 1992; the U.S. population dependent on alcohol (ages 12 and older) from 1991 to 1993 reflected a non-significant fluctuation from 9.6 million, to 7.9 million, to 8.6 million for those years; and the estimated number of people who became regular drinkers in each year increased from the early 1960s until the late 1970s. The number of new regular users, defined by the U.S. Public Health Service as people who drink alcohol once a month or more, peaked at 3.4 million in 1977, and since the 1980s, the number has remained at over 2 million new regular drinkers each year. Young adults age 18–25 are the most likely to report heavy alcohol use, which is defined as drinking five or more drinks per day on each of five or more days in the last 30 days.[33] Men at all ages are more likely then women to drink and report current heavy alcohol use; heavy drinking was reported by 5 percent of the population age 12 or older. Drinking rates for females tend to be more closely related to the rates for males in the 18–29 age groups, with gender difference becoming more pronounced with increasing age; and, rates in younger cohorts in general exceed rates for older cohorts.[34]

Regarding adolescents, alcohol is the drug used most often among high school seniors. "Although most high school seniors cannot legally buy alcoholic beverages, 90 percent of them had tried alcohol, compared with 64 percent who had tried cigarettes and fewer still who had tried other drugs."[35] The rate of alcohol use is likely to be higher among dropouts, and dropout rates differ among racial and ethnic groups. For example, dropout rates are higher than average among Native Americans and Hispanics and lower than average for Asian Americans; dropout rates for blacks and whites are comparable.[36] In a comprehensive study of the use of alcohol and other substances among American secondary school students, college students, and young adults from 1975 to 1991 it was found that, despite the fact that it is illegal for virtually all high school students and most college students to purchase alcoholic beverages, experience with alcohol is almost universal among the 88 percent of the high school seniors who have tried it, and active use is widespread.

Most important, perhaps, is the widespread occurrence of occasions of heavy drinking, measured by the percent reporting five or more drinks in a row at least once in a prior two-week period—among the high school seniors this statistic tends to be 30 percent, and among the college students it is about 43 percent. Since 1980, the monthly and daily prevalence of alcohol use among seniors has gradually declined; however there remains a quite substantial sex difference among high school seniors in the prevalence of occasions of heavy drinking (e.g., 21 percent for females versus 38 percent for males in 1991). This difference tends to be diminishing as well. Among college students, there is a significant difference among males and females in terms of their alcohol use with males drinking more. "For example, 52% of college males report having five or more drinks in row over the previous two weeks vs. 35% of college females."[37]

Alcohol abuse, alcohol dependence, and adverse consequences of drinking are less prevalent among individuals 65 and older than among those who are younger.[38] The percent of whites, blacks and Hispanics who are heavy drinkers does not differ significantly[39]; however, it is important to note that studies of alcohol abuse, alcohol dependence, and adverse consequences of drinking among racial and ethnic minorities have been sharply criticized for assuming that a given group is homogeneous.[40] "Developments in the field of ethnic and racial relations in the past several decades demand that interethnic variations be taken into consideration when examining alcohol-related questions. Such considerations would include assessment of ethnic identification, culture retention, incorporation of mainstream culture, and whether individuals are foreign-born or native-born. Because individual members of an ethnic group differ in the degree to which they objectively and subjectively identify with that group, it cannot be assumed that group membership is an adequate measure of ethnicity."[41] In terms of absolute numbers not controlling for population size, of the 10.9 million current heavy drinkers [in the United States] 81 percent are white, 9 percent are black, and 9 percent are Hispanic. About 1 percent of the current heavy drinkers are Native Americans, Asian/Pacific Islanders, and other groups.[42]

THE ALCOHOLIC: THEORIES AND PERSONALITY CHARACTERISTICS

Alcoholism is the most common form of addiction, and the typical drug addict is an alcoholic, not a street junkie.[43] Like most addictive substances, no single factor and no combination of multiple factors have been presented to predict which individuals will become alcohol abusers or dependent on the substance.[44] "Studying the factors that influence drinking is important in understanding how alcohol use and alcohol problems develop. Investigation of factors associated with drinking behavior can also shed light on the ways in which alcohol-related problems may be prevented and controlled."[45] The following information is a selective overview of theories and research associated with alcohol, utilizing a framework developed by Schuckit.[46]

Psychological factors include cognitive processes that include thinking, attention, and memory, and affective factors such as feelings and attitudes. One popular theory related to the motivation to drink is the tension-reduction hypothesis.[47] This theory suggests that alcohol is used to relieve tension caused by stressful life events. "The purported effect of alcohol on tension as it might relate to alcoholism can be broken down into two parts: the first consists of the hypothesis that alcoholics, when compared to [nonalcoholics], may have different baseline levels of anxiety, and the second part relates to the possible effects that alcohol might have in differentially decreasing levels of tension for alcoholics."[48] While many individuals think that alcohol helps them relax after a stressful day, there is little evidence that the use of alcohol in this manner causes alcoholism. In spite of a lack of evidence linking this theory to alcoholism, it is still a useful approach toward understanding the reasons for alcohol use, abuse, and dependence. Other psychological approaches that address issues of reinforcement and explain why people begin drinking, drink abusively, or remain alcoholics include receiving peer approval, enhancing or altering social interactions, changing levels of consciousness, decreasing the pressures of work, providing the opportunity to feel powerful and independent, and, blotting out unhappy memories or dampening stress response.[49]

Transactional theories are another approach used to explain the problem. Generally, it is assumed that poor communication may be responsible for initiating alcohol use and the progression to alcoholism and that levels of communication become more disordered as alcohol intake increases. It has been noted that alcoholism is the result of interaction in which the individual and the family use drunkenness and helplessness as an excuse for such behavior.[50]

The psychodynamic approach implies that alcohol is a reinforcing agent that helps the alcoholic fulfill some need, such as decreasing self-centered, narcissistic drives,[51] fulfilling a need for self-destructive punishment,[52] or addressing latent homosexuality.[53] Other theories under this rubric view alcohol use as a defense mechanism or protection against low self-esteem,[54] a means contributing to the achievement of power, and/or a way of generating care and dependence.[55] Personality theories tend to reflect no one personality type specific to the development of alcoholism, and the range of personality types of alcoholics is no different from that found in the general population,[56] but even for this statement an exception can be found. Antisocial personality disorder, for example, has been frequently associated with alcoholism. It has been "hypothesized that heavy drinking occurs not as alcoholism but as part of the antisocial picture, just as drug abuse, a high rate of divorce, accidents, and death by homicide can be seen in individuals with an antisocial picture."[57] Other psychological factors commonly associated with alcoholism include high levels of anxiety in interpersonal relations, emotional immaturity, ambivalence toward authority, low frustration tolerance, low self-esteem, feelings of isolation, perfectionism, guilt, compulsiveness, angry overdependency, sex-role confusion, an inability to express angry feelings adequately, narcissism, defiance, grandiosity, and resentment.[58]

A second major category of theories relates to sociocultural factors that have been used to study the historical aspects of alcohol abuse, compare how different societies view and respond to alcohol problems, and observe adaptive strategies used by individuals who have alcohol-related problems or who drink in the context of interpersonal relations.[59] Such factors are "typically defined as the impact of the environment, where environment is broadly interpreted to include not only the physical and social setting, but also the interpersonal behavior of others, including peers and family members. [The influence] can take many forms, and as with psychological processes, different factors have different effects on different people at different times. Also like psychological processes, social processes do not occur in isolation from other influences that motivate drinking."[60] It has been noted that "sociocultural theories can relate to drinking practices, drinking problems, or alcoholism . . . [they] serve as an impetus for theory formation and research but rarely, if ever, definitively answer questions."[61] Group norms, peer influences,[62] and expectancies about the effects of alcohol[63] influence drinking behavior. The effects of the home environment, including the influences of the family, on drinking behavior and the development of alcohol dependency, including childhood adjustment problems to later alcoholism, have been perhaps the most frequently studied social influence.[64]

Cultural theories relate alcohol use to the attitudes and behavior of a particular society or subgroups within a society.[65] Issues of parental child-raising practices[66]; social mobility, and access to opportunities (e.g., jobs and income),[67] as well as sex and work role expectations, particularly for women,[68] all fall into this category.

Biological factors show that "alcoholics have many body-functioning abnormalities [a finding that is] not surprising considering the ubiquitous effects of alcohol on the body and the damage done through chronic alcohol intake and dietary neglect."[69] Issues of biochemical effects, including sugar and carbohydrate metabolism dysfunction, food allergy, and other similar approaches to explaining alcoholism, are under investigation and speculative.[70] One factor, however, that has been receiving considerable investigation is genetics, which reveals the familial nature of alcoholism.[71] "Evidence of genetically transmitted vulnerability for alcoholism exists. Much of the evidence has arisen from adoption studies, but additional support for potential genetic contributions is found in research on markers of inherited susceptibility . . . twin studies suggest that the interaction between genetic and environmental influences is implicated in certain drinking behaviors."[72] Finally, it has been noted that "of all the variables studied, genetic factors were the easiest to investigate and have yielded findings of importance in establishing one element in particular of the many responsible for the final alcoholic picture."[73]

ALCOHOL USE AND CULTURE

Alcohol is a cultural artifact; the form and meanings of drinking alcoholic beverages are culturally defined, as are the uses of any other major artifact. The form is usually explicitly stipulated, including the kind of drink that can be used, the amount and rate of intake, the time and place of drinking, the accompanying ritual, the sex and age of the drinker, the reason for drinking, and the behavior proper to drinking. How a society socializes drunkenness is as important as how it socializes drinking.[74]

Each culture can be regarded as having a range of behavior that is integral to the culture.[75] In attempting to explain social organization and its relation to alcohol use, Bales used four attitudes to describe the use of alcohol. In some cases, societies exist which show an almost pure form of one of the attitudes. A combination of attitudes within a society also exists, and also a number of societies, as part of the process of social change, are in a state of transition between one attitude, or combination of attitudes and another. Regarding the attitudes:

The first calls for complete abstinence. For one reason or another, usually religious in nature, the use of alcohol as a beverage is not permitted for any purpose. The second might be called a ritual attitude toward drinking. This is also religious in nature, but it requires that alcoholic beverages, sometimes a particular one, should be used in the performance of religious ceremonies. Typically the beverage is regarded as sacred, it is consecrated to that end, and the partaking of it [is] a ritual act of communion with the sacred. . . . The third can be called a convivial attitude toward drinking. Drinking is a "social" rather than a religious ritual, performed both because it symbolizes social unity or solidarity and because it actually loosens up emotions which make for social ease and good will. This is what is often called "social drinking." The fourth type seems best described as a utilitarian attitude toward drinking. This includes medicinal drinking and other types calculated to further self-interest or personal satisfaction. It is often "solitary" drinking, but not necessarily so.[76]

The utilitarian attitude, essentially self-oriented, has been used to describe the patterns of alcohol use and abuse among the Irish, specifically, in terms of everyday use, to get rid of a hangover, to quiet hunger, to release sexual and aggressive tensions.[77] The ritual attitude defines the acceptable use of alcohol as largely restricted to religious functions. Jewish drinking and sobriety have been used as an example.[78] The convivial attitude is a mixture of the first two: it includes some ritual components that symbolize social solidarity, such as standing "shouts" or exchanging cups of sake, and some utilitarian components, such as the expectation of "good feeling" as a result of drinking. Bales considered that wherever convivial drinking "is found highly developed it seems to be in danger of breaking down toward purely utilitarian drinking."[79]

In general, "cultural attitudes predominately ritual or abstinent seem to be associated with a form of drinking highly integrated with other cultural characteristics and consistent throughout a given culture. Utilitarian attitudes, on the other hand, seem to be found mainly in modern, complex societies, in which both attitudes and drinking behavior are pluralistic and at times inconsistent. Convivial attitudes manifest themselves in a wide range of forms. In some cases they seem to be predominately integrative and associated with a low rate of alcoholism."[80]

Alcohol Use among Jewish People

It has been widely thought that the rate of alcohol abuse and alcoholism among Jewish people, in comparison to other ethnic and national groups, is low. Most of the studies on which this assumption is based "have been done in an attempt to understand the pattern of moderate drinking amongst Jews in the Diaspora (i.e., countries other than Israel), within the framework of a generally permissive attitude towards alcoholic beverages."[81] Research during the past decade suggests, however, that drinking patterns and problems tend to change as individuals interact with people of other religious or cultural backgrounds that stress different drinking norms.[82] Thus, in a study of alcohol use among undergraduate college students at 72 colleges in the United States in 1984 and 1985,[83] little difference was found between Jewish students and others in terms of alcohol-related attitudes and behavior. The study points to the significant degree of assimilation among Jewish people as a possible factor for the finding.

Historically, alcohol-related problems among Jews were unknown in Palestine during the British mandate period prior to the establishment of the state of Israel in 1948.[84] Factors such as the shared sense of mission to establish the state, a high level of motivation and pioneering spirit, and austerity provided controls on excessive alcohol-drinking behavior. "Social drinking habits, which were brought from countries of exile, were neglected or diminished within the context of the conscious change in the lifestyle of the immigrants."[85] This pattern of behavior appears to have held throughout the 1950s and up to the 1960s, when the controls mentioned before became less influential.

During the various waves of immigration to Israel, certain groups, especially from North Africa and Middle-Eastern countries, brought with them social drinking habits acquired in their countries of origin. Adaptation difficulties due to the breakage of patriarchism during the adjustment to the new modern country, sometimes turned a formerly moderate drinking habit into pathologically excessive drinking. A change of status due to a redefinition of the socioeconomic status of the head of the family, who had to compete in a society having a far different educational, social and economic level than that of his original society in his country of origin, causes economic difficulties. In addition to these, the tension of day to day life in Israel, under pressure from outside the country, from hostile states as well as from within [in terms of] Israel's highly competitive society, has hastened the tendency for [people] to fall back on drink as an escape mechanism.[86]

In addition to this group of Jewish people, excessive alcohol users existed among survivors of the Holocaust, who drank in order to cope with problems of adjustment and to escape from loneliness and the horrors of the past and its memories.[87]

During the 1970s, a different pattern of alcohol-related behavior emerged in Israel—a movement away from moderation and a generally pejorative attitude to one reflecting a greater acceptance of alcohol as a substance affecting the nature of interaction of people on an individual and group basis. Drinking became a "status symbol" and a "trademark of being worldly."[88] Several other factors also directly contributed to a spread of "hedonistic alcohol use" that promoted problems of abuse and alcoholism in the country. After the Six-Day War in 1967, there was a rise in the country's standard of living; and large numbers of volunteer workers from Western countries, who viewed alcohol as a means of pleasure and fun, influenced other young people in the country with whom they sought companionship. During the 1970s, a gradual change in values and norms developed in Israel. Personal motivation became dominant at the expense of human values, and Israeli society tried to be a society "like all societies." In the process of transition, it became difficult to maintain the moderate level of alcohol use that had characterized the isolated Jewish community in the Diaspora and in the period of the establishment of the state.[89]

Israel, to a major extent, has adopted Western culture and values, including its attitudes and behavior toward alcohol use. Since 1990, for example, the number of pubs throughout the country has increased from 100 to 2,000 in response to the growing demand for alcohol among veteran citizens, particularly the young, and from immigrants from the former Soviet Union. Another indicator of the rise of alcohol use in Israel is driving behavior. In 1992, the country's Highway Safety Administration of the Ministry of Transportation reported that 4–5 percent of road accidents were caused by drunk drivers, as compared to less than 2 percent during the previous year. Government officials cite the influx of Russian immigrants, a people with high levels of alcoholism, as a major factor in this growing problem, but they also point out that young Israelis are "emulating Western habits and are taking to the bottle. This, together with a lack of experience behind the wheel and a show of 'macho bravado,' appears to be contributing to an increase in fatal accidents."[90] This situation resulted in a law enacted in 1991 banning young people from driving between 1 A.M. and 5 A.M.; however, the legislation was repealed a year later as ineffective.[91]

University Student Alcohol Use: Patterns and Problems

The college or university is more than an institutional mechanism that provides opportunities for higher education, career development, and personal advancement; it is one of the primary means a society has to transmit cultural values and behavior through social interaction.[92] Research has been conducted to understand drinking among collegiate populations, document its frequency, and identify the consequences of negative drinking patterns, such as disruptions in personal relationships, problems with authority figures, impaired academic performance, fighting, and, physical or property damage.[93] Most studies have been done, however, with divergent theoretical and operational definitions that obfuscate understanding the extent of the problem. For example, the reported prevalence of students abusing alcohol ranges from such extremes as 6 percent to 72 percent.[94] Studies have reported at least occasional alcohol use by over 90 percent of the college students in the United States,[95] with consumption rates for the majority of student alcohol users ranging from one to ten drinking occasions per month and one to five drinks per occasion.[96] Confronted with such a range of numbers and facts, it is understandable why policy and program personnel involved with prevention and treatment of alcohol-related problem behaviors have difficulty addressing the issue. From information available, it is clear that there is no single factor explaining why a college student uses and/or abuses alcohol. Reasons that are commonly cited include the need to socialize, peer group pressure, escape from negative feelings or emotions, or simply getting drunk for the "fun of it."[97] It has been found that while most students drink to amplify positive affective conditions, problem drinkers also seek to escape negative ones or to use intoxication as an opportunity to express socially inappropriate behavior.[98]

Attitudinal and personality characteristics often found associated with problem drinking include lowered impulse control, greater proneness to deviant problem behavior, lower expectations of academic success, and greater value placed on independence than on academic achievement.[99] According to Jessor and Jessor,[100] a combination of personality characteristics with environmental and behavioral factors appears to best explain problem drinking. "Within this model, alcohol abuse is viewed as a behavioral pattern of problem-prone individuals likely to engage in other forms of deviant behavior as well. . . . Thus, the research on personality points to the importance of non-alcohol factors in understanding problem drinking. Furthermore, these factors, termed 'commonalities,' are thought to underlie other forms of substance abuse as well."[101]

The social context of peers, family, and environment is another important factor in considering drinking among college students. Studies have shown that the influence of social context is stronger than that of personality factors in predicting the initiation of, and involvement in, problem-drinking behavior patterns.[102] Moreover, from a review of relevant literature, it has been concluded that "among social context variables, peer influences have outweighed the effects of family and environment. . . . Young problem drinkers appear to have weaker ties to parents and are more oriented to peers, who provide influential models for their heavier alcohol use. In a study of a college population, [it has been demonstrated] that the influence of peers upon heavy drinking [is] far greater than that of other environmental and family characteristics."[103]

Alcohol Patterns and Problems among College Students of Singapore and Israel

Alcohol abuse is a worldwide problem; consequently, cross-cultural studies are important in identifying those behavioral patterns and environmental influences that are common to all alcohol users as separate from those factors that are culturally unique. The analysis that follows is based on one such effort, which includes three studies of university student alcohol patterns and problems conducted in Singapore (1988)[104] and Israel (1986, 1993),[105] utilizing a similar research methodology and a valid and reliable questionnaire that was originally designed by Engs and Hanson[106] and modified for use outside the United States. For discussion purposes, each study population is presented in terms of its own unique, alcohol-related characteristics and then compared on selected dimensions of the information collected.

In Singapore, the questionnaire was mailed to 1,848 students who were chosen by means of a stratified random sample methodology. Factors such as students' ethnicity, academic discipline, and year of study were addressed in the sample selection process. A usable response rate of 63 percent (N = 1,160) was achieved. Sixty-six percent (767) of the respondents were Chinese, 11 percent (121) were Malays, and 16 percent (185) were Indians. Approximately 7 percent (87) of the respondents were of other ethnic groups. Forty-seven percent (544) were men, and 53 percent (616) women. The largest group (29 percent) of the students was from the arts and social sciences; 24 percent were from the natural sciences; 14 percent (164) from engineering; 11 percent from business administration; and 22 percent from other departments.

In the Israeli study,[107] the questionnaire was distributed to 1,274 preparatory and undergraduate students. Instead of mailing the questionnaire, as in the Singapore study, students were asked to complete the instrument in class. Of the respondents, 92 percent were Jewish; 1 percent were Muslim; less than 1 percent (8) were Christians; and 6 percent (79) considered themselves atheists or agnostics. Fifty percent were men, and 50 percent were women. The largest group of students (29 percent) was from the social sciences and humanities; 8 percent were from the natural sciences; 27 percent from technology; 9 percent from medicine; 6 percent from nursing and physiotherapy; and 21 percent from the *mechnia* (college preparatory program). The sample of 1,274 students represented 16 percent of the overall student population of 8,200. A similar, unpublished study was conducted earlier in 1986 with a smaller cohort of 185 students at the same university.[108] A comparison of results, including factors of sex, alcohol preference, and a four-nation (Singapore, Israel, the United States, and Australia) comparison of selected problem behavior among drinking students, appears in Tables 4.1, 4.2, and 4.3 at the end of this chapter.

Multiple theories, conjectures, hypotheses, and correlates may be used to explain the alcohol-related patterns and problems of university students from Singapore, Israel, the United States, and Australia; it appears, however, that culture is a major factor affecting the decision to use and abuse alcohol. For Singapore students the findings reveal that, in consonance with other Asian groups, they use less alcohol than other ethnic populations. It appears that the content of their cultural values, traditions, attitudes, and beliefs; the degree to which they are socialized to their native culture; and the processes of acculturation that minimize family conflicts, role identity problems, and alienation are a bulwark against excessive alcohol use and problem behavior.[109] In Singapore, excessive drinking and related problems are viewed as being "disgraceful," not only for the individual but for the entire family. The stigmatization of such behavior, therefore, has been culturally ingrained, resulting in lower patterns of alcohol use.[110] Youth and young adults are not encouraged to drink, and adults drink only on festive occasions. Drunkenness is frowned upon in Chinese society.[111]

Compared to Singapore, other countries tend to have a more permissive attitude toward alcohol use and abuse. While there may be policies and legal sanctions regarding excessive drinking and potentially dangerous behavior (e.g., driving while intoxicated), the degree of enforcement in most countries is far from ideal, as evidenced by the data presented—for example, a comparison of those who reported driving a car knowing they had had too much to drink and those who indicated they had been arrested for drunk driving.

Another important dimension of college student alcohol use is gender differences, the extent to which college men and women are similar or different with regard to alcohol use patterns.[112]

Differences have been consistently reported in the literature regarding the consumption, motivations for, and consequences of men's and women's alcohol use. . . . Traditionally, there are encouragements for men's drinking and constraints upon women's drinking. . . . Yet, as sex role stereotypes become less rigid [e.g., in modern Western countries and those adopting western values, such as Israel], trends toward greater drinking among collegiate women might be anticipated as normative pressures against women's drinking relax somewhat.[113]

Singapore and, to a lesser extent, Israel (as compared to countries such as the United States and Australia) have the advantage of addressing alcohol problems from a preventive perspective rather than from a crisis situation. In these two countries, cultural patterns do not (yet) reflect excessive use or reliance on alcohol. For this reason, preventive strategies would appear to be a good public investment for them. Such strategies include education in the schools, restrictions on advertising for legal psychoactive substances (e.g., alcoholic beverages and cigarettes), and developing a societal orientation and a sense of peer pressure, especially for young people, that do not condone the use of alcohol and the accompanying negative behavior associated with it.[114]

In contrast, in the United States and Australia alcohol has penetrated many patterns of daily living, including those of work and leisure. In these societies, impacting the dominant values orientation and culture-related habits of people is a formidable challenge for those responsible for shaping and moving their countries toward a positive, productive, and healthy future.[115]

ALCOHOLISM: CASE EXAMPLES

The Case of W

W was 53 years old when his family finally convinced him to come for treatment. He had been drinking heavily for the last 23 years and was in very bad physical shape. According to him, he had been born to a relatively wealthy, middle-class family. His father used to drink occasionally but never got really drunk; his mother also used to sip cocktails at parties but nothing more.

When W finished high school, he started working as a distributor of cosmetics. It was a good life; he usually drove around visiting different shops and meeting female cosmetics experts, with whom he had several affairs. Finally, he married a woman he had known for years who was in no way connected to the cosmetics business; nevertheless, he continued to have his affairs with women connected with his business. With his wife, he had two daughters and one son, leading a relatively normal life and doing well economically. W used to drink socially, sometimes entertaining customers, sometimes at parties, but never too much or too often.

At age 30, the life of W changed abruptly when his wife was rammed by a truck while driving the family car. His son died in the traffic accident, and his wife sustained a severe injury to her spine that caused permanent paralysis of her legs, leaving her confined to a wheelchair and bed. Her character and relationship to W changed much as a consequence of the accident. W accused his wife of having caused the accident and was very depressed by the death of his son; nevertheless, he felt obligated to take care of his paralyzed wife. In order to alleviate his depression he started to drink. At the beginning, he would drink one or two glasses at night to cope with the stress at home, and with his depression and to be able to sleep. Gradually, he started increasing the amount he drank every night and after a few months he was drinking about half a bottle a day, which was affecting his ability to function, but he carried on with his work and living with his family. He continued this pattern of alcohol use for a few years, occasionally trying to reduce the amount he drank. Sometimes he would succeed especially during the week; however, on weekends he would return to a pattern of excessive alcohol use because he could not cope with his situation. He continued having extramarital affairs, but he now found justification for this action, since his wife could not have sexual intercourse due to her physical condition.

At age 40, his sex drive started to deteriorate, probably due to his heavy drinking. He consulted a physician, who advised him of the effects of alcohol and recommended that he go for treatment. W refused, claiming that if he quit drinking he would probably commit suicide. The physician recommended a visit to a psychiatrist, but W refused, believing that he was not crazy and that he was coping with the situation. Using large quantities of prescribed vitamins, his condition improved for a while, but his business was deteriorating, his customers complaining of his heavy alcohol smell and errors. The state of his affairs contributed to his depression, causing him to drink even more heavily to cope.

One night, driving back home while severely intoxicated, he rammed his car into a tree. W lost consciousness and spent the night in his car until somebody found him in the morning. The police were called to the scene of the accident, and W was sent to the hospital, where he was diagnosed as having aspirated his own vomit. During his stay in the hospital for a few days, W received treatment for injuries and for the alcohol withdrawal syndrome he developed. Upon his departure from the hospital he claimed he would stop drinking and would return to a more normal life. W stayed sober for about two months until other problems caused him to start drinking again in order to cope. Finally, at the request of his family, W went for treatment of his problem with alcohol, but not until he had lost his business, he was no longer able to care for his wife, and his own physical condition had deteriorated to the point that he was suffering from liver cirrhosis (a very serious liver condition mostly caused by alcohol), polyneuropathy, lung emphysema, and cardiac problems. Also, he had difficulties in concentrating and sleeping and was severely depressed.

The usual detoxification treatment worked very well for W, and he received counseling immediately upon completion of this initial stage of the treatment process. With the help of antidepressant medication his condition improved. W has been sober and stable for the last year and a half, he restarted his business but was not able to improve his relation with his wife, who initiated divorce proceedings.

The Case of J

J was the fifth son of eight children in a low-income family; his father worked as a cleaner in a supermarket, and his mother took care of the family while occasionally cleaning houses of other people. J was the son of an alcoholic and was an alcoholic himself. He was 32 when he reached out for treatment.

The home environment for J was not a pleasant one. His father would return home in the evenings after having drunk heavily—he would beat the wife severely from time to time or rape her in front of all the children. The father had also raped two of his daughters and had attempted to rape J. When J was about seven or eight, he ran away from home. His father swore he would kill him upon his return, but, instead of doing that, he severely beat him.

The two daughters who had been raped took to the street and started working as prostitutes at an early age and would share their income with their mother, who had difficulty providing food for everybody with the low wages the father earned. The father did not spend much money on alcohol because most of the time he simply stole it from the supermarket where he worked.

J started drinking at age 11 in his own home. He would sip a few drops from a bottle his father would have in the house. At age 12, he was working in the streets, running errands for shopkeepers, and getting into trouble with the police as a result of small thefts and other misdemeanors. By the time he reached 15, J drank every day, was belligerent like his father, and tried to rape his youngest sister, who was 9 at the time. He could not rape her because she was protected by the mother, but nobody blamed him for the attempt since it was more or less "normal" behavior in the family.

Due to his alcohol use and poor eating habits, J was very thin and often ill. Without proper medical care he developed a chronic lung condition that caused him to cough, which he would control by drinking. At about age 20 J was drunk most of the time, slept in the streets, and lived off the money he would beg for and could squeeze out of his sisters, who continued working as prostitutes. One day he tried to snatch a purse from an old lady but was caught by the police and sent to jail. During his time there he did not drink, but upon his release he continued to do so. Once on the streets again, J was run over by a car and taken to a hospital with a broken leg and other injuries. While there a social worker started to treat him for his alcoholism. The treatment was not very successful because J was not terribly interested in quitting his use of alcohol. He regained some weight and left the hospital with a cast on his leg, which gave him appeal as a beggar. Through his begging this time he was making enough money to eat regularly and to buy the alcohol he needed. From his perspective things were going well, so much so that he decided to forgo any treatment at the hospital for his alcoholism and even put off the removal of his cast.

The next tragedy in the life of J occurred when one of his sisters was accidentally killed in a shoot-out between delinquents. Apparently, this event provoked a sense of guilt and sorrow in J for the loss of his sister, who he believed had needed his protection which he had not been able to provide. Finally, he decided to stop drinking and try to rebuild his life, beginning with treatment. He was referred for detoxification, and his cast was finally removed, leaving him with a deformity, because the bone had not been set properly. After detoxification, he was referred to an admission unit where he received shelter and three meals a day and was sent to learn a profession. He chose to learn electricity, which gave him a certificate stating that he could be an assistant electrician, enabling him to work in buildings or other places under supervision. Also, J started attending Alcoholics Anonymous (AA) meetings and became very active in that organization. Soon after his departure from the admission unit he got a job and rented a small flat, inviting his sister, still working as a prostitute, to live with him. In a sense, they established an alliance to help each other with their difficulties. The remainder of the family had disintegrated—the father died of liver cancer; the mother left the city, never to be heard of again; and the other brothers and sisters went their own ways with no further contact among them.

After six years had passed since he had received treatment and in spite of all the difficulties he had encountered in his life, J maintained his abstinence, had a stable job, and continued living with his sister.

NOTES

1. American Psychiatric Association (1994). *Diagnostic and Statistical Manual of Mental Disorders*. 4th ed. Washington, DC: American Psychiatric Association, pp. 195–196.

2. Ibid, p. 196.

3. Goode, E. (1989). *Drugs in American Society*. 3rd ed. New York: McGraw-Hill, p. 16.

4. Keller, M. (1986). The old and the new in the treatment of alcoholism. In D. Strug, S. Priyadarsini, and M. Hyman (eds.), *Alcohol Interventions*. New York: Haworth Press, pp. 25–25.

5. Hafen, B. (1977). *Alcohol: The Crutch That Cripples*. St. Paul: West, pp. 1–2.

6. Ray, O., and Ksir, C. (1990). *Drugs, Society and Human Behavior.* St. Louis: Times Mirror/Mosby, p. 151.

7. Spring, J., and Buss, D. (1979). Three centuries of alcohol in Britain. In D. Robinson (ed.), *Alcohol Problems*. London: Macmillian, p. 25.

8. Wilson, C. (1973). *Food and Drink in Britain*. London: Constable Press.

9. National Institute of Mental Health. (1972). *Alcohol and Alcoholism: Problems, Programs and Progress*. National Institute of Mental Health, National Institute on Alcohol Abuse and Alcoholism, PHS Publication No. (HSM) 72-9127, p. 1.

10. Strug, D., Pryadarsini, S., and Hyman, M. (eds.) (1986). *Alcohol Interventions: Historical and Sociocultural Approaches*. New York: Haworth Press, p. 1.

11. Levine, H. (1978). The discovery of addiction: Changing conceptions of habitual drunkenness in America. *Journal of Studies on Alcohol* 39, no. 1: 143–174.

12. Keller, p. 27; *Alcohol and Health* (1990). U.S. Department of Health and Human Services, Rockville, MD, p. 3.

13. Strug, Pryadarsini, and Hyman, p. 3.

14. Hafen, pp. 1–2.

15. Levine, H. (1984). The alcohol problem in America: From temperance to alcoholism. *British Journal of Addiction* 79: 109–119.

16. Strug, Pryadarsini, and Hyman, p. 4.

17. Lender, M., and Martin, J. (1987). *Drinking in America*. London: Macmillan.

18. Grant, B., Noble, J., and Malin, H. (1986). Decline in liver cirrhosis mortality and components of change. *Alcohol Health and Research World* 10 (Spring): 66–69; Goode, p. 127.

19. Burgess, L. (1973) *Alcohol and Your Health*. Los Angeles: Charles Publishing.

20. Goode, pp. 123–124.

21. Keller, pp. 26–28.

22. Desmond, E. (1987). Out in the open: Changing attitudes and new research give fresh hope to alcoholics. *Time Magazine,* November 30, p. 29.

23. U.S. Department of Health and Human Services. (1993). *Alcohol and Health*. DHHS Pub. No. (ADM) 281-91-0003. Washington, DC: Superintendent of Documents, U.S. Government Printing Office, p. xxix.

24. Harwood, H., Kristiansen, P., and Rachal, J. (1985). *Social and Economic Costs of Alcohol Abuse and Alcoholism*. Issue Report No. 2. Research Triangle Park, NC: Research Triangle Institute.

25. Grant, B., DeBakey, S., and Zobeck, T. (1991). *Liver Cirrhosis Mortality in the United States, 1973–1988*. NIAAA Surveillance Report No. 18. DHHS Pub. No. (ADM) 281-89-0001. Washington, DC.: Superintendent of Documents U.S. Government Printing Office.

26. U.S. Department of Health and Human Services. (1993). *Alcohol and Health*. DHHS Pub. No. (ADM) 281-91-0003. Washington, DC.: Superintendent of Documents, U.S. Government Printing Office, p. 238.

27. Dietz, P., and Baker, S. (1974). Drowning: Epidemiology and prevention. *America Journal of Public Health* 64, no. 4: 303–312; Patetta, M., and Biddinger, P. (1988). Characteristics of drowning deaths in North Carolina. *Public Health Report* 103, no. 4: 406–411; Plueckhahn, V. (1982). Alcohol consumption and death by drowning in adults. *Journal of Studies on Alcohol* 43, no. 5: 445–452.

28. Goodman, R., Istre, G., Jordan, F., Herndon, J., and Kelaghan, J. (1991). Alcohol and fatal injuries in Oklahoma. *Journal of Studies on Alcohol* 52, no. 2: 156–161; Smith, S., Goodman, R., Thacker, S., Burton, A., Parsons, J., and Hudson, P. (1989). Alcohol and fatal injuries: Temporal patterns. *American Journal of Preventive Medicine* 5, no. 5: 296–302.

29. Noble, E. (1978). *Alcohol and Health*. Rockville, MD: National Institute on Alcohol Abuse and Alcoholism; DeLuca, J. (ed.). (1981). *Alcohol and Health*. Rockville, MD: National Institute on Alcohol Abuse and Alcoholism; Crum, R., Muntaner, C., Eaton, W., and Anthony, J. (1995). Occupational stress and the risk of alcohol abuse and dependence. *Alcohol Clinical Experimental Research* 19: 647–655; Zobeck, T., Grant, B., Stinson, F., and Bertolucci, D. (1994). Alcohol involvement in fatal traffic crashes in the United States: 1979–1990. *Addiction* 89: 227–233; Leigh, J. (1995). Dangerous jobs and heavy alcohol use in two national probability samples. *Alcohol and Alcoholism* 30: 71–86; Lahelma, E., Kangas, R., and Manderbacka, K. (1995). Drinking and unemployment: Contrasting patterns among men and women. *Drug and Alcohol Dependency* 37: 71–82.

30. Desmond, pp. 29–30.

31. Cohen, R. (1992). *Drunk Driving: 1989 Survey of Inmates of Local Jails*. Washington, DC: Bureau of Justice Statistics Special Report.

32. Lender and Martin, p. 206; Gallup, G. (1980). *The Gallup Poll: Public Opinion 1979* (1986), *The Gallup Poll: Public Opinion 1985* (1987), *The Gallup Poll: Public Opinion 1986*. Wilmington, DE: Scholarly Resources; Fishburne, P., Abelson, H., and Cisin, I. (1980). *National Survey on Drug Abuse: Main Findings, 1986*. Rockville, MD: NIDA; Johnson, L. O'Malley, P., and Bachman, J. (1987). *Drug Use among American High School Students, College Students, and Other Young Adults: National Trends through 1985*. Rockville, MD: NIDA. Goode, pp. 123–125; Barringer, F. (1991). With teens and alcohol, it's just say when. *New York Times*, June 23, p. 1.

33. Rouse, B. (ed.) (1995). *Substance Abuse and Mental Health Statistics Sourcebook*. DHHS Publication No. (SMA) 95-3064. Washington, DC: Superintendent of Documents, U.S. Government Printing Office.

34. Grant, B., Harford, T., Chou, P., Pickering, R., Dawson, D., Stinson,F., and Noble, J. (1991). Epidemiologic Bulletin No. 27: Prevalence of DSM-III-R alcohol abuse and dependence: United States, 1988. *Alcohol Health Research World* 15, no. 1: 91–96.

35. U.S. Department of Health and Human Services, p. 21.

36. Bachman, J., Wallace, J., O'Malley, P., Johnston, L., Kurth, C., and Neighbors, H. (1991). Racial/ethnic differences in smoking, drinking, and illicit drug use among American high school seniors, 1976–89. *American Journal of Public Health* 81, no. 3: 372–377.

37. Johnston, L., O'Malley, P., and Backman, J. (1992). *Smoking, Drinking and Illicit Drug Use among American Secondary School Students, College Students, and Young Adults, 1975-1991.* Rockville, MD: NIDA; U.S. Department of Health and Human Services, pp. 21–22.

38. U.S. Department of Health and Human Services, p. 36.

39. Rouse, B. (ed.) (1995). *Substance Abuse and Mental Health Statistics Sourcebook.* DHHS Publication No. (SMA) 95-3064. Wahington, DC: Superintendent of Documents. U.S. Government Printing Office, p. 63.

40. Cheung, Y. (1990–1991). Overview: Sharpening the focus on ethnicity. *International Journal of Addictions* 25, nos. 5A & 6A: 573–579; Heath, D. (1990–1991). Uses and misuses of the concept of ethnicity in alcohol studies: An essay in deconstruction. *International Journal of Addictions* 25, nos. 5A & 6A: 607–628.

41. U.S. Department of Health and Human Services, p. 24.

42. Rouse, B. (1995), op. cit., p. 63.

43. Goode, p. 108

44. Ray, O., and Ksir, C. (1990). *Drugs, Society, and Human Behavior.* St. Louis: TimesMirror/Mosby, p. 156; Vaillant, G. (1983). *The Natural History of Alcoholism.* Cambridge: Harvard University Press; Schuckit, M. (1986). Etiologic theories on alcoholism. In N. Estes and M. Heinemann (eds.), *Alcoholism: Development Consquences and Interventions.* St. Louis: Times Mirror/Mosby, pp. 15–30.

45. *Alcohol and Health*, p. 129.

46. Schuckit.

47. Conger, J. (1956). Alcoholism: Theory, problem and challenge: II. Reinforcement theory and the dynamics of alcoholism. *Quarterly Journal of Studies on Alcohol* 17: 296–305; Cappell, H., and Herman, C. (1972). Alcohol and tension reduction: A review, *Quarterly Journal of Studies on Alcohol* 33: 33–64.

48. Schuckit, p. 16

49. Ibid., p. 17

50. Steiner, C. (1971). *Games Alcoholics Play.* New York: Grower Press.

51. Conger.

52. Ward, R., and Faillace, L. (1970). The alcoholic and his helpers; a system view. *Quarterly Journal of Studies on Alcohol* 31: 684–691.

53. Schuckit, p. 18.

54. McCord, J. (1972). Etiological factors in alcoholism: Family and personal characteristics, *Quarterly Journal of Studies on Alcohol* 33: 1020–1027.

55. Schuckit, M., Morrison, C., and Gold, E. (1983). Alcoholism in women: Some clinical and social perspectives. In M. Greenblatt and M. Schuckit (Eds.), *Alcoholism Problems in Women and Children.* New York: Grune and Stratton.

56. Schuckit, M. (1984). *Drug and Alcohol Abuse: A Clinical Guide to Diagnosis and Treatment.* New York: Plenum Publishing Corp.

57. Schuckit, p. 19; Robins, L. (1978). Sturdy childhood predictors of adult antisocial behaviour: Replications from longitudinal studies. *Psychiatric Medicine* 8: 611–622.

58. Denzin, N. (1987). *The Alcoholic Self.* Newbury Park, CA: Sage, p. 31.

59. Heath, D. (1976). Anthropological perspectives on the social biology of alcohol: An introduction to the literature. In B. Kissim and H. Begleiter (eds.), *The Biology of Alcoholism*, vol. 4. New York: Plenum Press.

60. *Alcohol and Health*, p. 136.

61. Schuckit, p. 20.

62. Jessor, R., and Jessor, S. (1975). Adolescent development and the onset of drinking: A longitudinal study. *Journal of Studies on Alcohol* 36: 27–51; Zucker, R., and Noll, R. (1982). Precursors and developmental influences on drinking and alcoholism: Etiology from a longitudinal perspective. In National Institute on Alcohol Abuse and Alcoholism, *Alcohol Consumption and Related Problems*. Alcohol and Health Monograph No. 1. DHHS Pub. No. (ADM) 82-1190. Washington, DC: Superintendent of Documents, U.S. Government Printing Office, pp. 289–327.

63. Marlatt, G., Demming, B., and Reid, J. (1973). Loss of control drinking in alcoholics, an experimental analogue. *Journal of Abnormal Psychology* 81, no. 3: 233–241; Zinberg, N. (1984). *Drug, Set, Setting: The Basis for Controlled Intoxicant Use*. New Haven, CT: Yale University Press; Goldman, M., Brown, S., and Christiansen, B. (1987). Expectancy theory: Thinking about drinking. In H. Blane and K. Leonard (eds.), *Psychological Theories of Drinking and Alcoholism*. New York: Guilford, pp. 181–226.

64. McCord, J. (1988). Identifying developmental paradigms leading to alcoholism. *Journal of Studies on Alcohol* 49: 357–362; Werner, E. (1986). Resilient offspring of alcoholics: A longitudinal study from birth to age 18. *Journal of Studies on Alcohol* 47, no. 1: 34–40; Drake, R., and Vaillant, G. (1988). Predicting alcoholism and personality disorder in a 33-year longitudinal study of children of alcoholics. *British Journal of Addictions* 83: 917–927; Zucker, R., and Gomberg, E. (1986). Etiology of alcoholism reconsidered: The case for a bio-psychosocial process. *American Psychology* 41, no. 7: 783–793; Barnes, G. (1990). Impact of the family on adolescent drinking patterns. In R. Collins, K. Leonard, and J. Searles (eds.), *Alcohol and the Family: Research and Clinical Perspectives*. New York: Guilford Press, pp. 137–161; *Alcohol and Health*. (1990). U.S. Department of Health and Human Services (ADM) 90-1656. Washington, DC: Superintendent of Documents, U.S. Government Printing Office, pp. 4–6.

65. Roebuck, J., and Kessler, R. (1972). *The Etiology of Alcoholism: Constitutional, Psychological, and Sociological Approaches*. Springfield, Ill: Charles C. Thomas.

66. Bacon, M. (1974). The dependency-conflict hypothesis and the frequency of drunkenness. *Quarterly Journal of Studies on Alcohol* 35: 863–876.

67. Morrison, C., and Schuckit, M. (1978). Locus of control in young men with alcoholic relatives and controls. *Journal of Clinical Psychiatry* 44: 306–307.

68. Schuckit, M., and Morrissey, E. (1976). Alcoholism in women: Some clinical and social perspectives. In M. Greenblatt and M. Schuckit (eds.), *Alcoholism Problems in Women and Children*. New York: Grune and Stratton.

69. Schuckit, 21.

70. *Alcohol and Health* (1993), pp. 147–159.

71. Ibid., pp. 61–77; Cotton, N. (1979). The familial incidence of alcoholism. *Journal of Studies on Alcohol* 40: 89–116; Schuckit, p. 21.

72. Cloninger, C., Bohman, M., and Sigvardsson, S. (1981). Inheritance of alcohol abuse. *Archives of General Psychiatry* 38: 861–868; Goodwin, D., Schulsinger, F., Hermansen, L., Guze, S., and Winokur, G. (1973). Alcohol problems in adoptees raised apart from alcoholic biological parents. *Archives of General Psychiatry* 28: 238–243; *Alcohol and Health* (1990), p. 5.

73. Schuckit, p. 27.

74. Mandelbaum, D. (1979). Alcohol and culture. In D. Robinson (ed.), *Alcohol Problems*. London: Macmillian, pp. 15–21; Heath, D. (1975). A critical review of ethnographic studies of alcohol use. In R. Gibbons et al. (eds.), *Research Advances in Alcohol and Drug Problems*, vol. 2. New York: Wiley; Vailliant, G. (1983). *The Natural History of Alcoholism*. Cambridge: Harvard University Press, pp. 58–63.

75. Benedict, R. (1935). *Patterns of Culture*. London: Methuen; Sargent, M. (1973). *Alcoholism as a Social Problem*. St. Lucia, Queensland: University of Queensland Press, p. 35.

76. Bales, R. (1959). The cultural differences in rates of alcoholism. In R. McCarthy (ed.), *Drinking and Intoxification*. Glencoe, IL: Free Press, p. 267.

77. Bales, R. (1962). Attitudes toward drinking in the Irish culture. In D. Pittman and C. Synder (eds.), *Society, Culture and Drinking Patterns*. New York: Wiley, p. 185.

78. Snyder, C. (1962). Culture and Jewish sobriety: The ingroup-outgroup factor. In D. Pittman and C. Snyder (eds.), *Society, Culture and Drinking Patterns*. New York: Wiley, pp. 188–225.

79. Bales, R. (1959). Cultural differences in rates of alcoholism. In R. McCarthy (ed.), *Drinking and Intoxification*. Glencoe, IL: Free Press, pp. 263–277.

80. Lollo, G., Serianni, E., Golder, G., and Luzzatto-Fegiz, L. (1958). Alcohol in Italian culture. Food and wine in relation to sobriety among Italian Americans. Monographs of Rutgers University Centre of Alcohol Studies, No. 3 New Haven, CT: Free Press; Sargent, p. 39.

81. Weiss, S., and Eldar, P. (1987). Alcohol and alcohol problems: Research 14. Israel. *British Journal of Addiction* 82: 227.

82. Greeley, A., McGready, W., and Theisem, G. (1980). *Ethnic Drinking Subcultures*. New York: Praeger; Engs, R., Hanson, D., and Isralowitz, R. (1988). Drinking problems among Jewish college students in the United States and Israel. *The Journal of Social Psychology* 128, no. 3: 415–417.

83. Engs, R., and Hanson, D. (1985). The drinking patterns and problems of college students. *Journal of Alcohol and Drug Education* 31, no. 1: 65–83.

84. King, A. (1961). The alcohol problem in Israel. *Quarterly Journal of Studies on Alcohol 22: 321–328.*

85. Weiss and Eldar, p. 229; Shuval, R., and Kraslowsky, D. (1963). A study of hospitalized male alcoholics. *The Israel Annals of Psychiatry and Related Disciplines* 1: 277–292.

86. Weiss and Eldar, p. 229

87. Shuval and Kraslowsky; Weiss and Eldar, p. 229.

88. Weiss and Eldar, p. 229.

89. Ibid.

90. Sudilovsky, J. (1992). Teenage drinking. *Jerusalem Post,* October 1, p. 1B.

91. Marcus, R. (1993). Drunken driving accelerates throughout the country. *Jerusalem Post,* January 1, p. 9.

92. Wechsler, H. (1996). Alcohol and the American college campus. *Change,* July–August: 20–26; Gfroerer, J., Greenblatt, J., and Wright, D. (1997). Substance use in the U.S. college-age population: Differences according to educational status and living arrangement. *American Journal of Public Health* 87, no. 1: 62–65.

93. Berkowitz, A., and Perkins, W. (1986). Problem drinking among college students: A review of recent research. *Journal of American College Health* 35: 21–28; Wechsler, H., and

McFadden, M. (1979) Drinking among college students in New England. *Journal of Studies on Alcohol* 40: 969–996.

94. Wright, L. (1983). Correlates of reported drinking problems among male and female college students. *Journal of Alcohol and Drug Education* 28: 47–57.

95. Kozicki, Z. (1982). The measurement of drinking problems among college students at a midwestern university. *Journal of Alcohol and Drug Education* 27: 61–72.

96. Hughes, S., and Dodder, R. (1983). Alcohol consumption patterns among college populations. *Journal of College Student Personnel* 24: 257–264; Wechsler and McFadden; Maddox, G. (ed.) (1970). *The Domesticated Drug: Drinking among Collegians.* New Haven, CT: College and University Press.

97. Wechsler and McFadden; Maddox; Straus, R., and Bacon, S. (1953). *Drinking in College.* New Haven, CT: Yale University Press; Berkowitz, A., and Perkins, W. (1985). Gender differences in collegiate drinking: Longitudinal trends and development patterns. Paper presented at the Annual Meeting of the American College Personnel Association, Boston; Friend, K., and Koushki, P. (1984). Student substance use: Stability and change across college years. *International Journal of Addiction* 19: 571–575; Engs, R. (1977). Drinking patterns and drinking problems of college students. *Journal of Studies on Alcohol* 38: 2144–2156.

98. Berkowitz and Perkins, p. 23; Ratliff, K., and Burkhart, B. (1984). Sex differences in motivation for and effects of drinking among college students. *Journal of Student Alcohol* 45: 26–32.

99. Berkowitz and Perkins, pp. 23–24; Donovan, J., and Jessor, R. (1978). Adolescent problem drinking: Psychosocial correlates in a national sample study. *Journal of Studies in Alcohol* 39: 1506–1524; Donovan, J., Jessor, R., and Jessor, S. (1983). Problem drinking in adolescence and young adulthood: A follow-up study. *Journal of Studies on Alcohol* 44: 109–137.

100. Jessor and Jessor.

101. Berkowitz and Perkins, p. 24; Levinson, P., Gerstein, D., and Maloff, D. (eds.) (1983). *Commonalities in Substance Abuse and Habitual Behavior.* Lexington, MA: Lexington Books.

102. Berkowitz and Perkins, p. 24; Kandel, D. (1980). Drug and drinking behavior among youth. *Annual Review of Sociology* 6: 235–285; Zucker, R., and Noll, R. (1982). Precursors and developmental influences on drinking and alcoholism: Etiology from a longitudinal perspective. In *Alcohol and Health Monograph #1: Alcohol Consumption and Related Problems.* Rockville, MD: National Institute on Alcohol Abuse and Alcoholism.

103. Perkins, W. (1985). Religious traditions, parents, and peers as determinants of alcohol and drug use among college students. *Review of Religious Research* 27: 15–31.

104. Isralowitz, R. E., and Ong, T. H. (1988). Singapore: A study of university students' drinking behaviour. *British Journal of Addiction* 83: 1321–1323.

105. Isralowitz, R. (1987). Israeli college student drinking problems. Unpublished Report. Ben Gurion University, Beer-Sheva (Israel): Hubert H. Humphrey Institute for Social Ecology, Ben-Gurion University of the Negev; Isralowitz, R., and Peleg, A. (1993). Licit and Illicit Drug Patterns and Problems among University Students in Israel. Ben Gurion University, Beer-Sheva (Israel): Hubert H. Humphrey Institute for Social Ecology, Ben-Gurion University of the Negev.

106. Engs, R., and Hanson, D. (1975). Student alcohol questionnaire and the alcohol attitude questionnaire (Unpublished work). Bloomington: Indiana University and State University of New York at Potsdam.

107. Isralowitz, R., and Peleg, A. (1996). Israeli college student alcohol use: The association of background characteristics and regular drinking patterns. *Drug and Alcohol Dependence* 42: 147–153.

108. Isralowitz (1987).

109. Kim, S., McLeod, J., and Stantzis, C. (1992). Cultural competence for evaluators working with Asian-American communities: Some practical considerations. In M. Orlandi, R. Weston, and Epstein, L. (eds.), *Cultural Competence for Evaluators*. DHHS Publication No. (ADM) 92-1884. Washington, DC: U.S. Department of Health and Human Services, pp. 211–217.

110. Isralowitz and Ong.

111. Kua, E. (1987). A cross-cultural study of alcohol dependence in Singapore. *British Journal of Addiction* 82: 771–773.

112. Berkowitz, A., and Perkins, W. (1987). Research on gender differences in collegiate alcohol use. *Journal of American College Health* 36: 123–129.

113. Ibid., p. 123.

114. Eigen, L. (1991). *Alcohol, Practices, Policies, and Potentials of American Colleges and Universities*. DHHS Publication No. (ADM) 91-1842. Rockville, MD: U.S. Department of Health and Human Services.

115. Isralowitz, R., and Borowski, A. (1992). Australian university student alcohol behavior in perspective: A cross-cultural study. *Journal of Alcohol and Drug Education* 38: 39–42.

Table 4.1
Male and Female Student Drinking Patterns

	Singapore		Israel	
	Drinking (61%; N = 709)	Non-Drinking (39%; N = 451)	Drinking (74%; N = 946)	Non-Drinking (26%; N = 328)
Male	72% (390)	28% (154)	82% (522)	18% (117)
Female	52% (319)	48% (297)	67% (424)	33% (211)

Source: Isralowitz, R., and Peleg, A. (1993). Licit and Illicit Drug Patterns and Problems among University Students in Israel. Unpublished Report. Hubert H. Humphrey Institute for Social Ecology, Ben-Gurion University of the Negev.

Table 4.2
Drinking Student Alcohol Preferences
(percentage of drinking students who use the substance)

	Singapore	Israel
Beer	76%	84%
Wine	72%	83%
Hard Liquor	57%	73%

Source: Isralowitz, R., and Peleg, A. (1993). Licit and Illicit Drug Patterns and Problems among University Students in Israel. Unpublished Report. Hubert H. Humphrey Institute for Social Ecology, Ben-Gurion University of the Negev.

Table 4.3
Selected Consequences of College Student Alcohol Use

	Singapore[1] (N = 709)	Israel[2,3] (N = 135)[2] (N = 948)[3]	United States[4] (N = 2620)	Australia[5] (N = 155)
Hangover	27% (189)	36% (345)[3]	87% (2279)	72% (112)
Vomited	15% (107)	39% (53)[2]	82% (2136)	60% (93)
Driving after drinking	7% (53)	29% (279)[3]	74% (1938)	34% (53)
Driving and knowing they had too much to drink	2% (14)	20% (27)[2]	61% (1598)	24% (37)
Driving while drinking	<1% (3)	3% (26)[3]	59% (1558)	10% (15)
Arrested for drunk driving	<1% (1)	<1% (1)[2]	4% (92)	1% (2)
Thought they might have a drinking problem	2% (15)	5% (7)[2]	19% (510)	10% (16)
Cut a class after drinking	2% (14)	3% (27)[3]	22% (576)	18% (28)
Missed class because of a hangover	2% (14)	7% (67)[3]	40% (1046)	19% (29)
Criticized by date for drinking too much	2% (17)	15% (140)[3]	22% (588)	15% (23)

Sources: [1]Isralowitz, R. E., and Ong, T. H. (1988). Singapore: A study of university students' drinking behaviour. *British Journal of Addiction* 83: 1321–1323; [2]Isralowitz, R. (1987). Israeli college student drinking problems. Unpublished Report. Ben Gurion University, Beer-Sheva (Israel): Hubert H. Humphrey Institute for Social Ecology, Ben-Gurion University of the Negev; [3]Isralowitz, R., and Peleg, A. (1993). Licit and Illicit Drug Patterns and Problems among University Students in Israel. Unpublished Report. Ben Gurion University, Beer-Sheva (Israel): Hubert H. Humphrey Institute for Social Ecology, Ben-Gurion University of the Negev; [4]Engs, R., and Hanson, D. (1986). Age-specific alcohol prohibition and college students' drinking problems. *Psychological Reports* 59: 979–984; [5]Isralowitz, R., and Borowski, A. (1992). Australian university student alcohol behavior in perspective: A cross-cultural study. *Journal of Alcohol and Drug Education* 38: 39–42.

Chapter 5

Cocaine and Crack

HISTORICAL PERSPECTIVE

Sherlock Holmes "took his bottle . . . and hypodermic syringe and thrust the sharp point home, pressed down the tiny piston . . . with a sigh of satisfaction. . . . 'Which is it today,' he was asked, 'morphine or cocaine?' . . . 'It is cocaine . . . care to try it?' "[1] Sigmund Freud wrote, "I take very small doses of [cocaine] regularly against depression and against indigestion and with the most brilliant success."[2] He recommended cocaine as a local anesthetic, an aphrodisiac, and a means of treating depression, alcoholism, and morphine addiction.[3] By 1887, however, Freud had changed his mind on the merits of cocaine and wrote an article in which he said that cocaine was much more dangerous for public health than morphine.[4]

Categorized as a stimulant, cocaine use dates back more than 2,000 years to the Andes Mountains in South America. The Indians from the region (now Colombia, Peru, and Bolivia) still chew the leaves, which contain about 1 percent cocaine, to ward off fatigue and hunger, enabling them to work long hours without stopping. Evidence of the use of coca leaves has been found in a grave in Peru dating from about A.D. 500, and by A.D. 1000 the coca shrub was extensively cultivated in Peru. The ancient Incan civilization worshiped cocaine.[5] Despite efforts by Spanish invaders to stamp out its use, the coca leaf found its way to Europe, where its effects were studied by scientists and physicians.[6]

Isolated from coca leaves in about 1860 (the exact date is uncertain), cocaine became popular through Angelo Mariani, a French chemist, who developed a concoction known as Mariani's Coca Wine, which won praise from popes, kings, and presidents.[7] In 1885, the Parke-Davis Pharmaceutical Company noted that cocaine "can supply the place of food and make the coward brave" and called it a "wonder drug."[8] In 1886, a druggist by the name of John Styth formulated the syrup base for Coca-Cola by blending a whole leaf extract from the African kola nut, which is also a stimulant. Manufactured and marketed as medicine, Coca-Cola was touted as a temperance drink despite the fact that cocaine was still a key ingredient.

The manufacturer believed [the] product should not only be strongly associated with cocaine by the product name but also by the product package. Thus, the unique shape of the Coca-Cola bottle was originally intended to resemble the shape of the coca bean. In reality, the bottle shape resembles a cocoa bean because the production artists mistakenly used a cocoa bean, instead of a coca bean, as the model for the bottle design. In 1903, soon after the dangers of cocaine were publicized, the manufacturer of Coca-Cola removed cocaine from its formulation.[9]

Available in a large number of products for drinking, snorting, or injection,

all the elements needed to insure cocaine's outlaw status were present by the first years of the twentieth century: it had become widely used as a pleasure drug and doctors warned of the dangers attendant on indiscriminate sale and use; it had become identified with despised or poorly regarded groups—black, lower-class whites, and criminals; it had not been long enough established in the culture to ensure its survival; and, it had not, though used by them, become identified with the elite, thus losing what little chance it had for weathering the storm of criticism.[10]

The regulatory actions against the manufacture, sale, distribution, and use of cocaine eventually taken by the United States were at variance with the drug's wide acceptability. When the Harrison Act was used as a means of controlling drug addiction, during the Prohibition era of the 1920s in the United States, cocaine became less available and more expensive. Its use further declined in the 1930s with the introduction of inexpensive and easily available amphetamine substances and did not increase again until the end of the 1960s, when amphetamines became harder to obtain.[11]

During the early 1980s, cocaine abuse in the United States attained epidemic status. Estimates from the National Household Survey on Drug Abuse indicate that in 1994 there were 1.4 million active cocaine users in the United States. European countries, in comparison, did not experience dramatic increases in cocaine abuse but in the last few years there has been a progressive increase in the number of crack abusers.[12]

Crack

Until the late 1970s, the usual form of cocaine available on the street was cocaine hydrochloride, a salt form of cocaine that is usually sniffed (snorted) nasally or injected intravenously when mixed with water. Since the hydrochloride salt is quickly destroyed at high temperatures, it cannot be smoked unless it is in a freebase alkaloid form. Freebase cocaine is generally prepared by one of two ways. One method is to mix the hydrochloride salt with buffered ammonia; the alkaloidal cocaine is extracted from the solution using ether, and then the ether is evaporated to yield cocaine crystals. When heated, the crystals make a popping sound, and this characteristic sound is the origin of the term "crack." This form of cocaine is very pure and is generally called "freebase" on the street. The other method of producing freebase cocaine is to combine cocaine hydrochloride and sodium bicarbonate (baking soda) and heat the solution until a solid forms. The resultant pieces of the solid, also called "rock," when heated, release vaporized cocaine.[13] Since the mid-1980s, this has been the preferred method of production for smokable cocaine because it is simpler and safer than the ether extraction method. Today, most of the available crack cocaine in the United States has been produced in this manner.[14] For the last decade or so a lump, or rock, of crack cost about $10, which made it available to the poor.[15]

Cocaine and crack have become synonymous with the so-called "war on drugs." In 1982, the U.S. government allocated $200 million for a major initiative it thought would mark a turning point in the battle against drug violations and crime. Only seven years later, the government was promising $2.2 billion to finance its "war." Newspapers and magazine articles at that time reported the crack situation as follows:

Gangs that run the crack business, more fiercely armed and violence-prone than traditional racketeers, intimidate whole communities. In city after city, police report a startling rise in shootings of innocents struck by stray bullets . . . the criminal justice system, struggling to cope with crack-related crime, lacks energy and resources for everything else. And the numbing cost of more police, courts and especially prisons sucks away funds from education, health, housing and infrastructure . . . promiscuous sex in crack houses has become a powerful factor in the spread of AIDS. Overdoses, injuries and other health emergencies related to crack increased ten-fold from 1985 to 1987. The burden has pushed many urban clinics and hospitals to the brink, threatening all patients. The popularity of crack among women drags children into the drug problem on a scale never seen before. Intensive care for damaged babies born to crack-addicted women already costs $2.5 billion a year. Florida estimates it must spend $700 million to get the 17,500 crack babies born in 1987 ready for kindergarten. Everywhere, crack has generated an ugly wave of child abuse whose victims will lay heavy claim to social services the rest of their lives.[16]

In 1990, it was noted that at least 375,000, or 11 percent, of all newborns in the United States had been exposed to drugs in utero. Crack cocaine was the primary addiction of pregnant women.

Many of these babies start their lives with serious handicaps . . . they are likely to be born prematurely . . . more likely to have hydrocephaly (water on the brain), poor brain growth, kidney problems and apnea (when babies suddenly stop breathing) . . . they are also more likely to have suffered an infarct of the brain—similar to a stroke. . . . [As these children develop they have been found to be] either extremely irritable or very lethargic, have poor sucking abilities that hamper feeding and irregular sleep patterns . . . they may be hyperactive, slow in learning to talk and have trouble relating to other people.[17]

Unlike heroin, crack is popular with women. When they abuse it, they devastate their children as well as themselves . . . such a child [has been described] as a mere patch of flesh with a tangerine-sized head and limbs like splinters. Intensive hospital care for each crack baby costs about $90,000. That translates to $190 million a year in New York. For the nation, the figure is $2.5 billion. . . . [Probably] the most profound damage of crack may be to social values. Crack dealing involves more adolescents than the heroin trade ever did, offering them money enough to realize the most alluring teen-age fantasies—clothes, jewelry, cars, guns, power . . . [in response] vigilantism has begun to flare.[18]

According to the best estimates in the late 1980s, as many as 2.4 million Americans tried crack; but contrary to the myth of instant and total addiction, less than half a million used it once a month or more. Even among the current users, there are more occasional smokers than chronic abusers.[19] The irony of this situation is that it is somewhat parallel to an earlier cycle of cocaine use that occurred around the turn of the century: early acceptance as benign, a growing awareness of its dangers and side effects, and, finally, regulatory measures taken to control it. It has been suggested that the public is now in the second stage of this recurring cycle.[20]

TRENDS

In many major population centers throughout the United States, the number of cocaine users appears to be stable or on the decline especially in terms of cocaine-related deaths and toxicology mentions. Nevertheless, cocaine and crack continue to account for sizable proportions of total drug emergency department mentions. In most cities, cocaine (and crack) remains a major—if not the most commonly reported—illegal drug dealt with in emergency situations by medical personnel. As much as 20 percent or more of the cases treated are caused by cocaine and crack use. The following are highlights of the cocaine situation in the United States as reported by the National Institute of Drug Abuse.[21]

Use Patterns: The oldest age groups tend to make up the largest and fastest growing percentage of cocaine related deaths, emergency room visits and treatment interventions suggesting "a generally aging population suffering increased health consequences." These data support field reports that cocaine is increasingly acquiring a negative image among youth: their involvement in the cocaine scene appears limited largely to sales and distribution, often involving gangs. . . . Combinations [of use] include crack plus tobacco in a joint (called "bazookas" in Chicago), marijuana joints or "blunt" cigars laced with crack (called "geek joints" in Atlanta, "diablitos" or "primos" in Chicago, "oolies" in Boston, and "woolies" in New York) and PCP plus crack (called "spaceballs") in New York). In New York, "crisscrossing" involves sequentially inhaling lines of cocaine HCL and heroin. . . . Smoking (usually crack) remains the most reported [means of using the drug] . . . however, smoking may be declining, while intranasal use may be increasing among [hospital] admissions . . . inhaling cocaine HCL may be becoming more common among suburbanites and in association with the arts, entertainment, and club scenes. . . .

Although cocaine remains the most prevalent drug in arrestee urinalysis data, the percentages of cocaine-positive findings have generally declined [over time]. Many of the declines, especially among the younger adults, were offset by increases in marijuana rates.

Multisubstance Use and Shifting Use Patterns: Smoking (usually crack) remains, by far, the most reported primary route of administration among primary cocaine treatment admissions [and] . . . intranasal use . . . remains the most common mode among active recreational users not in treatment. . . . Mode of administration is often correlated with gender, race/ethnicity, age and other characteristics. For example, in [certain cities] smoking is more common among females than among males and among African-Americans than among whites or Hispanics. . . . [Also], in many cities, cocaine is even more of a problem as a secondary drug of abuse than as a primary drug. Alcohol and marijuana continue to be the most frequently reported secondary and tertiary substances of abuse among primary cocaine admissions.

Demographics:

(Age) Despite the growing evidence of an aging cocaine-using cohort, it is important to note that some youth are still initiating use . . . especially in conjunction with marijuana. . . . [Available] mortality figures for cocaine generally show decedents to be well over the age of 30. . . . Similarly, the rates of cocaine [emergency department] mentions per 100,000 population by age group continue to indicate an aging pool of cocaine users. . . . Treatment demographics, like the mortality and ED figures, . . . support the notion of an aging cocaine-using population.

(Gender) While female cocaine users account for between 17 and 30 percent of the mortality demographics in major cities, males account for the majority of deaths, emergency department mentions and cocaine treatment admissions . . . in all locations throughout the United States.

(Race/Ethnicity) In areas where cocaine mortality figures are available, the racial/ethnic distribution often differs strikingly. . . . In San Diego, [for example], 52 percent of the decedents were white, 23 percent were African-American (an overrepresentation), and 25 percent were Hispanic; whites also predominated in treatment admissions. In Los Angeles, African-Americans represented more than half of the decedents and treatment admissions. . . . One possible explanation for this difference is that emergency departments treat a greater diversity of populations than do treatment programs. However, this phenomenon warrants further investigation, especially since it is not as consistently noted among heroin users.

Law Enforcement Data:

(Availability, Price, and Purity) Crack and cocaine hydrochloride (HCL) prices and purity have increased [or at least remained stable in most major population centers]. [In certain locations such as Chicago and Seattle] stiff competition . . . has resulted in marketing schemes such as "2-for-1" sales and free-sample giveaways . . . . Vials for packaging crack are increasingly being replaced by cellophane wrappers in New York City and by small plastic bags (known as "CDs") in Philadelphia.

(Crime and Violence). . . . Ethnographic data [from Atlanta, Minneapolis and Denver] show an increase of crack sales and abuse as well as drive-by shootings and carjackings among members of several gangs, which results in an increase of random violence and deaths. Drug-related homicides . . . in areas where crack is sold . . . continue to involve handguns and gang activity.

THE COCAINE USER: PERSONALITY AND OTHER CHARACTERISTICS

Many users of illicit drugs experience psychological dependence, physical dependence, and drug addiction as a result of the harmful substances they use. Cocaine, however, is not addictive in the same way that heroin and other opiates are; nevertheless, its potential for creating psychological dependence may be high, especially in the form of crack.

The symptoms of heavy opiate (especially heroin) use give rise to the concept of drug addiction. In some ways the symptoms of cocaine use mimic those of heroin use, but in other ways they do not. Frequent cocaine users are clearly characterized by compulsive use and psychological dependence. They are not characterized by the physical dependence of heavy opiate use. The distress associated with cocaine withdrawal is suggested to be more psychological than physiological.[22]

Different drugs are used in different ways. For example, the effects related to drug use are slowest for swallowing and sniffing and fastest for smoking and injection. Intravenous injection deposits drugs directly into the brain. Drugs inhaled in smoke are absorbed by blood vessels in the lungs and carried to the brain. The physical effects of cocaine are felt within 30 seconds after intravenous injection. The high from smoking cocaine begins within 8 seconds and is more intense and short-lived than from other modes of use. While cocaine can be sniffed or snorted, smoked, swallowed, or injected, it has been found that about 90 percent of those who use cocaine sniff or snort the substance, 30 percent tend toward smoking it, and 10 percent swallow the drug.[23] Among the total household population age 12 or older who have used an illegal substance, 33 percent had used marijuana and/or hashish in their lifetimes; cocaine is the second most common substance tried. About 12 percent of the illicit drug users have tried cocaine, and about 2 percent have tried crack. These figures compare with the less than 2 percent who have ever used heroin.[24] In terms of the amount of money spent on illegal drugs, even with the decreased pattern of use currently reported, cocaine ranks first. In 1990, the Office of National Drug Control estimated that drug consumers in the United States spent $18 billion for cocaine compared to $12 billion for heroin, $9 billion for marijuana, and $2 billion for other drugs.[25]

COCAINE: THE LATIN AMERICAN PLAGUE

The primary location for coca leaf, the source for cocaine hydrochloride and crack, is Peru's Upper Huallaga Valley. In terms of total production, it has been estimated that Peru produces 63 percent, Bolivia 26 percent, and Colombia 10 percent of the coca, which, according to 1990 estimates, totaled 310,170 metric tons. "In Peru, Bolivia and Colombia, an estimated 1 million people, including farmers and laborers, grow coca leaves and process and export cocaine products; in Peru, as many as 60,000 families are thought to depend on coca growing for their livelihood; and in Bolivia, an estimated 350,000 to 400,000 people, 5–6 percent of the population, are directly employed in the cocaine industry."[26] At the growing and harvesting stage, those involved are simple farmers and rural laborers who are out to earn an income by growing a crop long consumed without great danger. "They know full well they are breaking the law, but that is unfortunately common in societies with large informal sectors that have been forced by government rules to operate outside the law."[27] The income from the cocaine industry grew in the late 1970s and early 1980s. Such a rise was associated with the deep economic troubles of Bolivia and Peru in terms of government deficits and rampant inflation. A vicious cycle was created for these two countries when the price for coca leaf soared, while the legal economy was in a state of decline. In order to temporarily hide conditions, the Bolivian and Peruvian governments created massive overemployment in the government and in loss-making, state-owned enterprises. With the major populations centers no longer able to absorb migrants from the overcrowded and resource-poor highlands, "it could be argued that without legal job alternatives [poor people], from the highlands had little choice but to move to the coca-growing regions, greatly increasing the labor available to grow coca."[28]

Cocaine production has proven to be a profitable undertaking for the farmer and trafficker; nevertheless, it has had serious negative effects on Latin American societies. The problems include *direct economic costs*—governments have been forced to spend more of their scarce resources on the police, courts, and military; *indirect economic costs*—legal industry has been displaced, there has been a loss of control over economic policy, and governments' inability to tax the cocaine industry has forced them to tax legal industries more heavily; *social costs*—while less prevalent than in the United States, cocaine consumption in Latin America is on the rise, causing an increase in social problems; *ecological costs*—poisonous chemicals are used in the production of cocaine and vast quantities are dumped into rivers. For example, turning coca leaves into coca paste requires the use of kerosene, sulfuric acid, and sodium bicarbonate; making a cocaine base out of a coca paste requires sulfuric acid, potassium permanganate, and ammonia hydrochloride; and turning the cocaine base to powdered cocaine necessitates the use of ethyl ether, acetone, and hydrochloric acid. Of course, other substitute chemicals can be used in the process; however, for each kilogram of cocaine, between 65 and 130 gallons of kerosene and smaller amounts of the other chemicals are required.[29] Also, the growing of coca on steep slopes causes erosion and destruction of forests; and *political costs*—the cocaine industry undermines fragile social democracies and weakens the ability to maintain law and order as well as curb corruption and terrorism.[30]

The need to bring cocaine to its principal market, the United States, has generated a considerable amount of ingenious illegal import activity. For example, one courier had a half pound of cocaine surgically implanted under the skin of each of his thighs. The cocaine was divided into four, one-square-inch packages of one-quarter pound each. Cocaine has been carried across the border in Arizona on the backs of mules or horses or on foot. Variable amounts of cocaine have been containerized and shipped out of Ecuador with such products as shrimp, cacao, and bananas. Tons of cocaine have been shipped from Venezuela to Miami inside concrete fencing posts; in false-bottomed metal boxes labeled as toilet seats and bathroom sinks; in counterfeit bottles of Pony Malta de Bavaria; in 55-gallon drums of guava pulp with the cocaine in plastic packets inside the fruit; in cardboard boxes packed with canned fruit stuffed with cocaine; in anchovy cans shipped from Argentina; in stuffed teddy bears, Peruvian handicrafts, and cans marked asparagus. Panamanian cocaine smugglers have developed a new technology that combines cocaine with vinyl to produce a material that has been used in making luggage and sneakers. The cocaine is separated from the vinyl after reaching its destination. Cocaine has been smuggled in suitcases hidden behind interior panels of airplanes; hidden in a secret tank within the fuel tank of a cabin cruiser; packed in one kilogram lots and placed inside a plastic pipe bolted to the bottom of a banana boat docked in Bridgeport, Connecticut, harbor. It has been sewn into the interior roof of a family stationwagon and transported during a family vacation; in a false compartment in the floor of a mobile home; and in the gas tank of a car equipped with a baffle that made the left side a separate compartment.[31]

COCAINE AND CRACK ADDICTION: CASE EXAMPLES

The Case of M

M was 35 years old when he came for treatment. He had been using cocaine for the last four years and had succeeded in ruining his career, losing his family and house, and having a stroke. Although his case is somewhat extreme, it illustrates some of the problems encountered when treating cocaine addiction.

M was the youngest of three children of a well-to-do couple who owned a food distribution center in a small town on the East Coast of the United States. Academically capable, M majored in business administration at a university. During his time there he used marijuana and beer in moderate amounts for social purposes with his friends. Upon graduation, he married a girl he had met in college and went to work with his father—his income was relatively high, and he had the money to buy what he wanted, including a house.

In spite of his good fortune, M experienced problems with his wife that affected his self-confidence. In response, he began to frequent nightclubs with his friends, who introduced him to cocaine. His first experience with the substance was a positive one that gave him the feeling that he could outperform everybody at the party and that he "belonged" in that kind of life. He bragged about his experience to his wife, who took the occasion to criticize and deride him. In response, M bought a large amount of cocaine, and, to impress some of his friends, he organized a men's party, inviting them to share the substance. Most of his friends did not share his interest in cocaine, and soon he felt alone with the need to relate to a new reference group. He was soon using several grams a day.

Over time, M began neglecting his work obligations, and his father was very upset about it. After several conversations, he disclosed to his father that he had been using cocaine, and his father requested he stop using the substance, or their association would be terminated. M tried, halfheartedly, to stop, but he did not succeed; his father terminated their association, gave him some money, and moved him out of the business.

By this time M had two children and his wife to support. Since he was not working, he started using the money he had received from his father to support the family and buy cocaine. The money was quickly used up, and, soon after, his wife filed for a divorce on the grounds that he was neglecting his family obligations and using drugs. From this action, she acquired the house, custody of the children, and alimony. Since M could not afford the alimony, his father took up the responsibility to support his grandchildren and to prevent his son from being prosecuted. M soon left his hometown and returned to the city, where he had personal contacts who he believed would be supportive and provide him with cocaine. Without money, M took up selling drugs to his friends to support his need for cocaine. He also had to use the cheapest forms of cocaine, including crack.

One day while smoking he felt a strange feeling in his head and fainted. When he woke up, he was in the emergency ward of a public hospital, where his condition was diagnosed as "mild stroke," most probably caused by drug use. M recovered quickly but not without a slight impairment in his left hand. Identified by the police as a first-time offender whose infraction was a relatively small one, he received a suspended sentence with the recommendation that he go for treatment.

Cocaine withdrawal syndrome is mostly psychological. There are no clear biological symptoms and signs, such as in alcohol or opiates withdrawal. The problem with cocaine, unlike alcohol or opiates, is that patients may stop using the substance without feeling any particular discomfort; however, after a few hours or days, they begin to feel empty and depressed, lack motivation, and believe that life without cocaine is worthless. Psychological treatment aimed at fighting the depression is difficult, and, since antidepressants do not help, the patients soon find themselves looking for more cocaine in order to alleviate their state of psychological discomfort. In the case of M, there was not much motivation for treatment, his ego strengths had been weakened before his use of cocaine, his wife and children had left him, and he had no job or sources of income. He had nowhere to turn and nowhere to return, making treatment difficult. Eventually, his father came to his rescue, providing him with basics, including a room for sleeping and an account at a cafeteria so that he could eat. Also, his father was ready to cover the cost of treatment if M was willing to undergo the process; however, on the advice of a therapist he was not prepared to provide his son with any money in cash.

M started therapy, including individual and group intervention methods in an ambulatory facility, since he refused to be admitted in a live-in center. After two months without any progress, he started to use cocaine again. Once again, he obtained the cocaine with money he received from selling drugs to friends. Having abandoned treatment, he left town in a van, traveling and doing his thing—using whatever form of cocaine he could get hold of and peddling it to make a living. In response to this situation, his father severed contact with him, and his communications with his brother and sister ended as well. M ceased trying to contact his children after his ex-wife threatened to call the police if he ever came near them while intoxicated, which was now his permanent status. Eventually, M was admitted to a psychiatric hospital in a state of paranoia probably due to cocaine. At the beginning of the stay there he tried to sever his penis, claiming that it was useless because he was not man anymore.

Psychotic episodes due to cocaine abuse are usually short-lived except if there is an underlying pathological condition such as schizophrenia, which probably existed in the case of M. The last heard about M was that he was still in the hospital and would probably stay there for some time since he was considered a danger to himself because of the attempted self-mutilation.

The Case of B

B was a well-known photographer of advertising models who owned his own studio. He married a much younger woman who tended to be jealous and insecure, especially when he had to work late hours with one of the models. They had no children because B considered himself too young at age 32 to have such responsibilities when there was so much for him to achieve. B worked very long hours, was chronically tired and tense, and believed he was losing his creativity. Some friends suggested that he try cocaine to improve his physical condition and restore his creative energies and emotional disposition.

B accepted their recommendation and started using cocaine on weekends with the belief that the substance could be used two or three days a week without harm or addiction. At the start of his cocaine use, B had lots of work and money, so buying cocaine was no problem. What B did not know was that people under stress soon find themselves using cocaine every day and that a psychological addiction tends to set in. Once he started using cocaine on a regular basis, he began losing weight, and his life became disorganized, so much so that his wife became very worried. At that point he decided the time had come for treatment.

An intelligent and sociable person with good verbal skills, B understood his problem. After about one year, during which time he had not used cocaine for six months, B decided that he was cured and that he needed to change his life, so he divorced his wife and took some partners into his business so that he could work less. He was so thankful for the treatment that he used his connections with the newspapers to have a story published about how he had been an addict and, thanks to the treatment he had received, how he had overcome the problem.

B disappeared from the treatment clinic and was not heard from for some time. After about two years he was seen on television in a program about sex addiction, telling people how he had been cured from his cocaine addiction only to become a sex addict; how he had been in treatment at a specialized clinic and how the efforts of the clinic's personnel had cured him of the problem. The last that was heard about B, from another addict under treatment, was that he had been attending meetings of Gamblers Anonymous—evidencing the psychological, rather than the physical, dimensions of the problem. Getting cured of cocaine addiction only to become addicted to something else is a rather common pattern of behavior.

NOTES

1. Doyle, A. (1938). The sign of the four. In *The Complete Sherlock Holmes*. New York: Garden City, pp. 91–92.

2. Taylor, N. (1949). *Flight from Reality*. New York: Duell, Sloan, and Pearce, p. 17.

3. Freud, S. (1974). Uber coca. In R. Byck (ed.), *Cocaine Papers*. New York: Stonehill, pp. 49–73.

4. Brain, P., and Coward, G. (1989) A review of the history, actions, and legitimate uses of cocaine. *Journal of Substance Abuse* 1: 431–451.

5. Antonil, C. (1978). *Mama Coca*. London: Hassle Free Press.

6. Goode, E. (1989). *Drugs in American Society*. New York: McGraw-Hill, p. 194.

7. Andrews, G., and Solomon, D. (eds.) (1975). *The Coca Leaf and Cocaine Papers*. New York: Harcourt Brace Jovanovich.

8. Perry, C. (1972). The star-spangled powder. *Rolling Stone*, August 17, p. 26.

9. Cornish, J., and O'Brien, C. (1996). Crack cocaine abuse: An epidemic with many public health consequences. *Annual Review of Public Health* 17: 260–261.

10. Ashley, R. (1975). *Cocaine: Its History, Uses and Effects*. New York: St. Martin's Press.

11. Ray, O., and Ksir, C. (1990). *Drugs, Society and Human Behavior*. St. Louis, MO: Times Mirror/Mosby, p. 129.

12. Cornish and O'Brien, pp. 262–263.

13. Jaffe, J. (1990) Drug addiction and drug abuse. In A. Gilman, T. Rall, A. Nies, and P. Taylor, (eds.), *The Pharmacological Basis of Therapeutics*. New York: Pergamon, pp. 522–545.

14. Cornish and O'Brien, pp. 259–260.

15. Ray and Ksir, pp. 134–135.

16. *New York Times*. (1989). Some war; meanwhile, crack undermines America. *New York Times*, (IE), September 24, p. 6.

17. Kantrowitz, B. (1990) The crack children. *Newsweek*, February 12, pp. 50–51.

18. *New York Times*. (1989). Crack: A disaster of historic dimension, still growing. *New York Times*, (IE), Editorial, May 28, p. 6.

19. Martz, L. (1990). A dirty drug secret. *Newsweek*, February 19, pp. 44–45.

20. Ray and Ksir, pp. 135–136.

21. National Institute of Drug Abuse. (1996). *Epidemiological Trends in Drug Use*, vol. 1. Rockville, MD: NIDA, pp. 13–14.

22. Bureau of Justice Statistics. (1992). Drugs, Crime and the Justice System: A National Report. Washington, DC: U.S. Department of Justice, p. 21.

23. Ibid., p. 24.

24. NIDA. (1991). *Highlights of the 1990 National National Household Survey on Drug Abuse*. Washington, DC: U.S. Department of Justice, Bureau of Justice Statistics, p. 27.

25. Bureau of Justice Statistics, p. 36.

26. Ibid.

27. U.S. Information Agency. (1992). *Consequences of Illegal Drug Trade: the Negative Economic, Political, and Social Effects of Cocaine in Latin America*, p. 6.

28. Ibid., p. 9.

29. Drug Enforcement Agency. (1991). *Coca Cultivation and Cocaine Processing: An Overview*. February, Table 2, p. 8.; Bureau of Justice Statistics, p. 40.

30. U.S. Information Agency, pp. 2–3.

31. Bureau of Justice Statistics, p. 45.

Chapter 6

Marijuana: Is It Really a War of Values and Special Interests?

HISTORICAL PERSPECTIVE

No illegal substance in the United States has generated more controversy and perhaps investigation in terms of impact on individual behavior and society than marijuana.

The marijuana, cannabis, or hemp plant is one of the oldest psychoactive plants known to humanity. It is botanically classified as a member of the Family Cannabaceae and the genus Cannabis . . . [which] grows as weed and cultivated plant all over the world in a variety of climates and soils. The fiber has been used for cloth and paper for centuries and was the most important source of rope until the development of synthetic fibers. The seeds (or, strictly speaking, akenes—small hard fruits) have been used as bird feed and sometimes as human food. The oil contained in the seeds was once used for lighting and soap and is sometimes employed in the manufacture of varnish, linoleum, and artist' paints. . . . The chemical compounds responsible for the intoxicating and medicinal effects are found mainly in a sticky golden resin excluded from the flowers on the female plants. . . . The plants highest in resin . . . grow in hot regions like Mexico, the Middle East, and India. . . . The three varieties are known as bhang, ganja, and charas. The least potent and cheapest preparation, bhang, is produced from the dried and crushed leaves, seeds, and stems. Ganja, prepared from the flowering tops of cultivated female plants, is two or three times as strong as bhang; the difference is somewhat akin to the difference between beer and fine scotch. Charas is the pure resin, also known as hashish in the Middle East. Any of these preparations can be smoked, eaten or mixed in drinks. The marijuana used in the United States is equivalent to bhang or, increasingly in recent years, to ganja.[1]

"Cannabis may have been cultivated as long as ten thousand years ago. It was certainly grown in China by 4000 B.C. and in Turkestan by 3000 B.C. It also has long been used as a medicine in India, China, the Middle East, Southeast Asia, South Africa and South America."[2] The earliest reference to cannabis is in a pharmacy book written in 2737 B.C. by the Chinese emperor Shen Nung. Referring to the euphoriant effects of the substance, he called it the "liberator of Sin." There were some medical uses, among which included "female weakness, gout, rheumatism, malaria, beriberi, constipation and absent mindedness."[3] By A.D. 1000, the social use of the plant spread to the Muslim world and North Africa; and in the region of the Middle East its use was associated with a religious cult that committed murder for political reasons. The cult was called Hashishiyya, from which the word "assassin" developed. Stories related to the substance involving intrigue, sex, and murder spread throughout Europe for centuries. French soldiers with Napoleon's campaign in Egypt used hashish, as did many other Frenchmen who worked for the government or traveled in the Near East during the nineteenth century. Also, during that time, hashish was used by writers like Baudelaire, Gautier, and Dumas as well as impressionistic artists. Among the descriptions of the experience is the following:

The intoxication will be nothing but one immense dream . . . at first, a certain absurd, irresistible hilarity overcomes you . . . after a few minutes the relation between ideas becomes so vague, and the thread of your thoughts grows so tenuous, that only your cohorts . . . can understand you . . . next your senses become extraordinarily keen and acute. Your sight is infinite. Your ear can discern the slightest perceptible sound, even through the shrillest of noises. . . . The strangest ambiguities, the most inexplicable transpositions of ideas take place. In sounds there is color; in color there is a music. . . . This fantasy goes on for an eternity. A lucid interval, and a great expenditure of effort, permit you to look at the clock. The eternity turns out to have been only a minute. . . . The third phase . . . is something beyond description. It is what Orientals call kef; it is complete happiness. There is nothing whirling and tumultuous about it. It is a calm and placid beatitude. Every difficult question that presents a point of contention . . . becomes clear. Every contradiction is reconciled. Man has surpassed the gods.[4]

A considerable amount of medical attention was given to cannabis from 1840 to 1900 recommending it for a variety of illnesses and discomforts. Among its recommended uses were as an analgesic (in the form of tincture of hemp—a solution of cannabis in alcohol taken orally); as a topical anesthetic for the mouth and tongue; and for problems and discomfort related to tetanus, neuralgia, dysmenorrhea (painful menstruation), convulsions, rheumatic and childbirth pain, asthma, postpartum psychosis, gonorrhea, and chronic bronchitis, for preventing migraine attacks, certain kinds of epilepsy, depression, asthma, rheumatism, gastric ulcer, and drug addiction, particularly of morphine and other opiate substances.[5] By 1890, the medical use of cannabis was on the decline. Among the reasons were that the potency of the preparations was too variable, and the invention of the hypodermic syringe in the 1850s made opiates more effective in pain relief since hemp products are insoluble in water and cannot be easily administered by injection. Also, synthetic drugs like aspirin, chloral hydrate, and barbiturates, which are chemically more stable, became attractive for medicinal purposes in spite of their disadvantages.

In the 1930s, marijuana received considerable negative attention—specifically, that the substance "would cause users to go crazy and become violent; men would rape and kill under the influence, and women would become promiscuous. Publications from the period had titles such as 'Marijuana—Sex-Crazy Drug Menace,' 'Marijuana—The Weed of Madness,' and 'Marijuana: Assassin of Youth.' Today these supposed effects receive no attention even in the most vigorous anti-marijuana polemics."[6] "Almost no observer argues that, in a single episode of use, marijuana generates psychosis, violence, or sexual 'excess' in the typical user. These issues are simply no longer the focus of controversy. . . . While the acute effects were emphasized in the 1930's, it is the chronic effects that have become the center of attention today."[7]

Generally speaking, little attention was given to marijuana during the early part of this century. There were references, however, linking the substance to Mexican Americans. "The prejudices and fears that greeted peasant immigrants also extended to their traditional means of intoxication—smoking marijuana." Also,

police officers in Texas claimed that marijuana incited violent crimes, aroused a "lust for blood," and gave its users "superhuman strength." Rumors spread that Mexicans were distributing the "killer weed" to unsuspecting American schoolchildren; and, sailors and West Indian immigrants were reported to have brought the practice of smoking marijuana to port cities along the Gulf of Mexico. In New Orleans, newspaper articles associated the drug with African-Americans, jazz musicians, prostitutes, and underworld whites. The "Marijuana Menace," as sketched by anti-drug campaigners, was personified by inferior races and social deviants.[8]

Curiously, in 1931, the commissioner of narcotics, Harry Anslinger, said that up to that year the Bureau of Narcotics file on marijuana was less than two inches thick[9]; yet the Treasury Department stated, "A great deal of public interest has been aroused by the newspaper articles appearing from time to time on the evils of the abuse of marijuana, or Indian hemp. . . . This publicity tends to magnify the extent of the evil and lends color to an inference that there is an alarming spread of the improper use of the drug, whereas the actual increase in such use may not have been inordinately large."[10]

The early 1930s were a turning point for marijuana; in fact, it is reasonable to say that the war on marijuana began at that time, with public opinion being shaped by Anslinger, who has been likened to J. Edgar Hoover in terms of conservative, staunchly anticommunist, law-and-order values and "idiosyncrasies" that were strongly imposed on their (i.e., Anslinger and Hoover) federal bureaucracies and personnel.

Anslinger did not believe in a public-health approach to drug addiction; he dismissed treatment clinics as "morphine feeding stations" and barrooms for addicts. In his view, strict enforcement of the law was the only proper response to illegal drug use; he urged judges to "jail offenders, then throw away the key." [It is interesting to note that] in his memoir, *The Murderers*, Anslinger confessed to having arranged a regular supply of morphine for "one of the influential members of Congress," who had become an addict. Anslinger's biographer believes that addict was Senator Joseph R. McCarthy.[11]

By 1935 there were 36 states with laws regulating the use, sale, and/or possession of marijuana, and by the end of 1936 all 48 states had similar laws. In 1937, congressional hearings were held, and Anslinger stated that "traffic in marijuana is increasing to such an extent that it has come to be the cause for the greatest national concern."[12] This position was precipitated by police reports, newspapers, and popular literature linking marijuana to violent crime, psychosis, and mental deterioration.[13] Among the statements were that marijuana makes the smoker vicious, with a desire to fight and kill, and that marijuana smokers are key suspects in horrible crime and perversion.[14] In spite of articles that contradicted this position (e.g., the chief psychiatrist at Bellevue Hospital in New York City said, "None of the assault cases could be said to have been committed under the drug's influence. Of the sexual crimes, there was none due to marijuana intoxication. . . . It is quite probable that alcohol is more responsible as an agent for crime than is marijuana."[15] Anslinger pressed on, and the film *Reefer Madness*, made as part of his campaign, was regarded as a serious attempt to influence public opinion and to shape policy.[16] Indeed, it did, and evidence reveals it was done based on heresy, little or no experimentation or reference to scientific undertakings, myth, and distortion of reality.[17] Why? Among the reasons were that the Great Depression made people sensitive and wary of any new and particularly foreign influences; lower-class Mexican Americans and African Americans who had initiated use of the drug made the drug even more dangerous to the white middle-class; the substance was associated with crime and murders committed by the cult Assassins.[18] This campaign lead to acceptance of the Marijuana Tax Act of 1937. "The general characteristics of the law followed the regulation by taxation theme of the Harrison Act of 1914. The federal law did not outlaw Cannabis or its preparations; it just taxed the grower, distributor, seller, and buyer and made it, administratively, almost impossible to have anything to do with [the substance]."[19] Once in place, the Marijuana Tax Act was credited with the immediate dramatic reduction of violent crimes committed under the influence of marijuana and the price of a marijuana cigarette, over a few years, increased 6–12 times to about a dollar.[20]

After the passage of the legislation, a number of significant events took place that contribute to further understanding the dynamics at play regarding marijuana use. Among the most significant were the findings by the New York Academy of Medicine in 1944 that marijuana impairs intellectual and physical functioning of an individual but does not affect the basic personality of the person, and over time those who have been smoking marijuana show no mental or physical deterioration that may be attributed to the substance. Strong reaction from the American Medical Association claimed that the New York study was too narrow and that sweeping and inadequate conclusions were drawn from an unscientific foundation that minimized the harm caused by marijuana use.[21]

As in all such reports and reactions to reports, there is little dispute over the facts, only over the interpretation. Since the LaGuardia Report (i.e., the New York Academy of Medicine's study which resulted in a book called Marijuana Problems by New York City Mayor's Commission on Marijuana) is in substantial agreement with the Indian Hemp Commission Report of the 1890s, the Panama Canal Zone reports of the 1930s, and the comprehensive reports in the 1970s by the governments of New Zealand, Canada, Great Britain, and the United States, in addition to the 1981 report to the World Health Organization and the 1982 report by the National Academy of Science to the Congress of the United States, it is likely that the conclusions of the La Guardia Report were and are for the most part valid.[22]

In the 1970s, the antimarijuana forces appeared to be on the defensive, especially since the drug had been decriminalized in 11 states making up a third of the nation's population. Fearing a growing epidemic was taking place in the nation, Senator James Eastland conducted a series of Senate subcommittee hearings on the *Marijuana-Hashish Epidemic and Its Impact on the United States Security.*[23] These hearings, in a manner similar to that used by Anslinger 40 years earlier, brought together witnesses and researchers who shared one factor in common: they had something negative to say about marijuana. "Any researcher who had conducted a study showing that marijuana was not harmful was not invited to deliver testimony. [And Eastland stated that] we make no apology . . . for the one-sided nature of our hearings—they were deliberately planned that way."[24] The claims, most of which were not able to stand up to retest validation, concluded that marijuana caused brain damage, massive damage to the entire cellular process, including chromosomal abnormalities, adverse effects on the reproductive process causing sterility and impotence, cancer, and a life of lethargy called the "amotivational syndrome." Eastland's response to the testimony and reports was that if the "cannabis epidemic continues to spread . . . we may find ourselves saddled with a large population of semi-zombies."[25]

In contrast to the biased and mostly inaccurate information presented at the Eastland hearings, Sussman et al. provide a detailed analysis of the negative consequences of marijuana. The results show that

the most well-confirmed danger from marijuana use is lung damage (and probably lung cancer). . . . A second potential negative consequence is that marijuana use appears to reduce the effectiveness of the immune system, although it may be a temporary reduction and may or may not be a medical concern among regular users. . . . Third, it apparently impairs biosynthesis of nucleic acids and proteins which may disrupt selective attention and long-term memory encoding if used over several years. . . . A fourth potential consequence includes pregnancy-related effects such as low birth weight and prematurity, although the data are equivocal. . . . Fifth, very high doses produce a toxic delirium (especially if eaten), the symptoms of which include confusion, agitation, disorientation, loss of coordination, and hallucinations. There have not been any reports of deaths from overdoses,[however]. . . . A sixth potential, but unconfirmed, consequence of chronic marijuana use is that it reduces one's motivation to accomplish goals. . . . [Seventh, marijuana] has been found to be associated with a lower sperm count; however, this association may be temporary. . . . An eighth consequence is that adult users report subjective difficulties. These difficulties, which may or may not have empirically observable behavioral or functional correlates, include impairment of memory, concentration, motivation, self-esteem, interpersonal relationships, health, employment and finances, safety, and pregnancy. . . . Ninth, marijuana use also has been investigated as a stepping stone drug. A number of studies indicate that marijuana users are at relatively high risk for use of other hard drugs and their related negative consequences. . . . A tenth potential consequence is that marijuana may be addictive. Psychological dependence (e.g., conditioning effects) appears to be more important than physical dependence regarding withdrawal of use. . . . Finally, [the substance] affects coordination that may place users at risk for accidents. THC [trans-delta-tetrahydrocannabinol] which is the primary psychoactive agent in marijuana] is found in the blood of more than 30% of fatally injured drivers, and more than 50% of persons stopped for reckless driving show detectable levels of marijuana, or marijuana and another drug, tested in urine.[26]

A substantial amount of evidence has accumulated about the relatively benign consequences of marijuana use. Additionally, the significant benefits of marijuana use in the treatment process for cancer, AIDS, and other serious illnesses are widely acknowledged and being addressed through such action as state legislation, for example, the overwhelmingly approved (California) Proposition 215—the Compassionate Use Act of 1996, which has made it possible for any "seriously ill" Californian to obtain marijuana upon the recommendation of a physician.[27] In spite of the body of knowledge available about marijuana and state-level actions being taken, federal opposition to marijuana use in any form has remained strong. In the wake of 215's passage and the Arizona legislative initiative that allows doctors to prescribe any drug for legitimate medical purposes and mandates treatment, not incarceration, for those arrested for illegal drug possession,[28] General McCaffrey (director of the White House's Office of National Drug Control Policy) began calling for "science not ideology" to settle the medical marijuana debate. McCaffrey has ordered a comprehensive National Academy of Science review of the literature on the subject, but the timing of the study leads many marijuana advocates to dismiss the measure as a tactic to delay any substantive reform of the issue. Even so, McCaffrey's call for more science is significant since it initiates a process that may prove that the benefits of marijuana outweigh the negative factors associated with its use. A similar review was conducted during the Carter administration, lending support to the medical use of marijuana; however, this conclusion was suppressed by government officials.[29]

Social, Political, and Economic Factors Leading to Policy Formation

The social, political, and economic factors associated with marijuana, including those related to the passage of the Marijuana Tax Act of 1937 and the Eastland congressional hearings in 1974, raise a number of interesting and somewhat puzzling questions. Among them is the dramatic shift of attitude of narcotics and government officials, including Anslinger, toward marijuana use in a very short period of time. Such a turnaround was certainly not based on well-documented and researched information. Regarding the link made between Mexicans and marijuana, themes of racism and national security may have been used to curb the influx of unwanted cheap labor. Since the early 1920s, Mexican immigration into the United States increased considerably, especially to the states bordering on Mexico. Mexican people were a cheap source of labor and were sought to develop large-scale agriculture in the South. Consequently, under pressure of both the Mexican government and large-scale farmers, Mexicans were not included in quota regulations.[30] Nevertheless, "led by patriotic organizations [like the] American Legion, small farmers and labor unions, a passionate and racist campaign started against Mexicans."[31] In an environment scarred by the Great Depression and driven toward unionism, the connection between Mexican people and other minority groups and violence and marijuana became an effective strategy to promote legislation and regulatory actions that dealt not only with marijuana (e.g., Marijuana Tax Act of 1937) but immigration and migrant farmworkers.[32]

In 1920, the Volstead Act brought about a total national Prohibition on the sale of alcohol.

The Volstead Act was passed because abstinence was identified with a prestigious and powerful group in American society. Prohibition failed because it was the powerful, prestigious middle class that abandoned abstinence as a legitimate and respectable way of life. Temperance ceased to be necessary to a respectable life; its symbolic connection with respectability was served. And lastly, the Depression loomed before the American public and the government, and relegalizing alcohol manufacture and sale brought with it the prospect of jobs and tax revenue.[33]

Marijuana was associated with underclass, marginalized populations labeled a threat to white, middle-class safety and law and order; nevertheless, it may have been seen as a potential source of competition for profits to be reaped by the alcohol industry and state and federal governments. The question that arises, especially now that the evidence is in on the cigarette industry, is to what extent he alcohol industry may have influenced government officials like Anslinger, Eastland, and others, as well as law enforcement personnel, to protect its interests and profits by restricting the availability of marijuana in America?

At the turn of the century numerous reports and personal experiences by physicians surfaced regarding the positive effects of marijuana for a range of illnesses. Parke-Davis Pharmaceutical Company, a leader in pharmaceuticals, recognized the importance of marijuana; yet; in spite of its practical applications and benefits the substance was removed from the public scene once it was labeled an illegal drug. With a cheap and relatively effective medicine out of the way, drug companies were compelled to research and develop synthetic substances to address the needs of America's unending appetite for ache and pain remedies. In the process, they acquired profits as well as a considerable degree of influence over the health care industry, including perhaps medical associations (e.g., the California Medical Association, which had failed to support Proposition 215). Put in other words, it appears that much was to be gained by the health care industry to have a useful, inexpensive drug like marijuana strictly regulated and, in fact, banished to the ranks of illegality.

Drug producers and dealers, too, may be thought of as an interest group with something to lose if a soft policy toward marijuana use prevailed. With government controls to limit production and accessibility, the cost of the substance to the user would rise, creating greater profit for those involved with its sale. "If increased drug prices are seen as a success story, then the increase in marijuana prices is the greatest success"[34]—not only for government applying this criterion as a successful outcome of its efforts but for those seeking higher profits from growing and selling the substance.

Any of the preceding descriptions of self-interest may have played a role in the formation of marijuana policy and, more importantly, the ways in which regulations have been interpreted by police and the judiciary. One additional factor is surely worth consideration—it involves the process of problem creation and elements of legitimation to control and preserve the resources, status, and power of individuals and their followers. The creation of a problem put before the public may have begun in the 1920s with scare tactics that marijuana use caused violent behavior, that its spread was a threat to national security, and that the substance had infiltrated the schools, putting the well-being of young people at risk. There was no well-documented evidence of these conditions, as noted in testimony before the House Ways and Means Committee regarding the Marijuana Act of 1937. Dr. W. C. Woodward, a physician-lawyer serving as a legislative counsel for the American Medical Association, argued "for less restrictive legislation on the ground that future investigators might discover substantial medical uses for cannabis" and that there was little evidence to support the contention that marijuana was harmful.[35] In his testimony, Woodward stated that newspaper accounts were not based on "competent primary evidence," and that the Bureau of Prisons had no evidence to show on the number of prisoners found addicted to marijuana; contrary to statements that schoolchildren were the great users of marijuana cigarettes, no evidence had been presented by the Children's Bureau to show the nature and extent of the habit among children, and that inquiry of the Children's Bureau showed that it had no reason to investigate the issue. A similar response was presented concerning the position of the Office of Education.[36] "His [i.e., Dr. Woodward's] objections to the quality and sources of the evidence against cannabis did not endear him to the legislators."[37]

Marijuana use came to be associated with people considered marginal to society, and Mexican Americans and African Americans became targeted as scapegoats for the problem. Also, there is much evidence that information was manipulated by government officials for use by the media—"saying bad things [by the press] about drugs is never questioned, and disconfirming information never requires revision of original claims."[38] Other means used to strengthen the government's policy toward marijuana included controlled congressional testimonies; denouncement of reports like those produced in New York for Mayor LaGuardia, as well as other professionally prepared studies on marijuana; the subjective application of law in terms of adjudication procedures such as minimum mandatory sentencing and the application of civil forfeiture statutes passed by Congress in the 1980s[39]; and the strong-arm tactics used by supporters of government-sponsored antidrug programs against those who questioned and challenged the effectiveness of efforts such as Drug Abuse Resistance Education Program (DARE).[40] In sum, the process of problem and people manipulation regarding marijuana use may have been used by Anslinger, Eastland, and others to promote their self-interests at the considerable expense and suffering of others.

TRENDS

Generally, patterns of marijuana use over the last 20 years or so do not indicate that government efforts have been successful in reducing or controlling the use of the substance. "The encouraging downturn in drug use of the early 1980s halted in 1985 [not just among adolescents but among college students and young adults as well]. . . . The use of marijuana, for example, fell from 37% in 1978 to 25% in 1984, a one-third decline, and daily marijuana use fell proportionally even more over the same interval, from 11% in 1975 to 5%; however, both declines halted in 1985."[41] In 1992, "among youth 12–21 years of age, controlling for differences in age composition, 26.5 percent of adolescent current [cigarette] smokers reported marijuana use in the previous 30 days."[42]

Since 1992, teenage marijuana use has grown considerably; by one measure it has doubled. "But that increase cannot be attributed to any slackening in the enforcement of the nation's marijuana laws. In fact, the number of Americans arrested each year for marijuana offenses has increased by 43 percent since Clinton took office. There were roughly 600,000 marijuana-related arrests nationwide in 1995—an all-time record. More Americans are in prison today for marijuana offenses than at any other time in our history. And yet teenage marijuana use continues to grow."[43]

In 1995, a study conducted by the Partnership for a Drug-Free America tracked attitudes toward drugs in 1994 among 8,520 children and 822 parents across the United States. It was found that teenagers were more tolerant about marijuana, and this trend was attributed, in part, to a glamorization of drugs in pop music, movies, and television shows and to an absence of national and community leadership in discouraging experimentation with drugs. Teenagers were found less likely to consider drug use harmful and risky and more likely to believe that drug use is widespread and tolerated and to feel more pressure to try illegal drugs than teens did just two years prior to the study. In response, an expert, Dr. Lloyd Johnston, described the resurgence as a case of "inter-generational forgetting" as adolescents who learned the dangers of drugs grew up and moved on. "Each new generation needs to learn the same lessons about drugs if they're going to be protected from them."[44] In another study conducted on substance use in the United States, it was found that the highest rates of past-month marijuana use were found among high school dropouts, particularly those living with parents, and college students not living with parents. Also, it was found that college students were not more likely than high school graduates to use marijuana.[45]

From the prevailing evidence, the culture of cannabis has grown. Among the reasons are more efficient agriculture, including new methods of harvesting and producing marijuana plants—the substance now is about 20 times more potent than what was on the streets in the 1960s and 1970s; the generation that laughed through *Reefer Madness* may be ignoring new findings about the nature of addiction and the effect marijuana has on memory, the lungs, and the immune system; and perhaps, because earlier messages about the dangers of marijuana were so over-heated and hyperbolic, serious research of recent years has not received attention or acceptance.[46]

Drawing from the National Institute of Drug Abuse (NIDA) report,[47] the following information relates to the patterns and problems associated with marijuana use:

Use Patterns and Multisubstance Use: "Blunts (Vega)"—gutted cigars refilled with mari-juana—remain entrenched in the culture of adolescents and young adults [throughout the United States]. . . . Marijuana tends to be used in combination with other substances, particularly alcohol and cocaine (usually crack) and, sometimes, phencyclidine (PCP). Some of the increase in adverse effects may be attributed to these other drugs. Neverthe-less, a substantial proportion of marijuana ED [hospital emergency department] mentions involves marijuana alone (21 percent in 1994). Among primary marijuana treatment admissions, alcohol is generally the most common secondary drug of abuse . . . however, in many cities . . . a sizable portion of marijuana admissions do not report another drug of choice. . . . Blunt smoking is frequently accompanied by alcohol consumption. In Chicago, youth often combine smoking blunts with drinking malt liquor. Another common weekend evening purchase is a package of blunts [cigars], razor blades to slit them open, and champagne. . . . "Blunts" smoked sequentially—one laced with mari-juana and the other with PCP—are called the "dream team." . . . Marijuana and PCP are frequently mixed with the combination called a "love boat" or "wets" or "lilies" . . . marijuana-cocaine combinations are referred to as "geek joints," "oolies," "diablitos," "primos," and "woolies" [depending on the city].

Demographics:

(Age): The 18–25 age group accounts for the highest national rate of marijuana ED mentions. Between the first halves of 1994 and 1995, however, marijuana ED rates apparently increased for all age groups (although the increase for the 12–17 group was not statistically significant at $p < 0.05$). . . . Youth are increasingly dominating the marijuana treatment demographics. In most areas, primary marijuana users are generally younger than primary cocaine or heroin admissions. The younger than 17 group now accounts for the highest percentages of marijuana admissions in [many cities throughout the United States].

(Gender): Males outnumber females nationally among marijuana ED mentions (2.4:1).

(Race/Ethnicity): Racial/ethnic distributions of primary marijuana treatment admissions vary across the country. Whites account for the largest proportions in nine areas (Atlanta, Boston, Chicago, Denver, Minneapolis/St. Paul, San Diego, Seattle, Texas, and the Washington/Baltimore [area]; African-Americans have the greatest representation in seven areas (Denver, Miami, Newark, New Orleans, New York City, Philadelphia, and St. Louis); and Hispanics are the modal group in Los Angeles.

Law Enforcement Data:

(Arrestee Data): Juvenile offenders primarily choose marijuana rather than harder drugs, in part because they participate in the distribution network for harder drugs. The number of marijuana arrests continues to increase. . . . In New York City, such arrests have been increasing since 1991 despite the decriminalization of possession of small amounts. In Boston, [for example], marijuana arrests accounted for 20 percent of all drug arrests in the first half of 1995, up from a low of 14 percent. . . . In Miami, marijuana criminal cases represent 33 percent of all drug cases.

(Availability, Price, and Quality): Wide availability [and potency] continues to be reported [throughout the United States]. Generally, marijuana may be purchased for as little as $40 per ounce (e.g., in Texas for the Mexican or domestically grown substance) and as much as $400–600 per ounce for high potency marijuana with a THC level of from 14–16%.

(Cultivation, Seizures, and Trafficking): Domestic cultivation, especially indoor hydroponics, continues to be reported in many areas. Colorado remains one of the leading States for indoor cultivation, but a large amount is also smuggled from Mexico. The Nation's largest indoor operation seizure so far in 1996 occurred in a Colorado cave. The second largest confiscation was in a private home in Miami. An increasing number of such hydroponic farms have been seized in Miami private homes. . . . Some Latin American marijuana, however, still enters Miami from Jamaica, the Bahamas, and other Caribbean transshipment points. . . . Trafficking patterns in Atlanta have shifted from coastal marine and air smuggling to complex indoor growing with hydroponics and domestic interstate shipments; however, Mexico remains a primary source, with Hispanic couriers and transporters being increasingly utilized. . . . At least 80 percent of the marijuana seized in the Seattle area is grown indoors. Many local growers are also reported in San Francisco. In Arizona, where marijuana is the most trafficked drug, foreign-grown marijuana is more prevalent in the southern and central areas, while domestically grown marijuana is more typically found in the higher elevations. . . . In Missouri, too, production is increasingly shifting to indoor operations, but many eradicated plants in Missouri are still grown in fields or on river banks. Much of the Missouri-grown marijuana is shipped out of State. . . . Intelligence in Texas suggests that previously active Colombian marijuana trafficking organizations are moving back into the marijuana market. Traffickers in Mexican marijuana in Texas are usually whites or Hispanics, while growers of domestic marijuana tend to be whites.

MARIJUANA USE: THE DUTCH EXPERIENCE

No country has received more attention than the Netherlands in terms of addressing the use of marijuana through liberal policy. After a period of "lenience" that began in 1968 and lasted for about eight years, the national government of the Netherlands revised the Dutch Opium Act in 1976, and, as a result, the most significant and talked about aspects of the changes made has been the de facto decriminalization of cannabis in small amounts.[48] Such de facto decriminalization, however, "was more the result of the absence of policy, and a response to already existing circumstances, than of any rational, well-considered action."[49] In this sense, the conditions underlying the formation of policy in the Netherlands and the United States tend to be similar; however, the results have been very different—one a "self-willed," lenient approach to soft drugs, and the other a controlled, prohibitive way of managing the use of marijuana.

Drawing from the research of Cohen,[50] a number of findings evidence the result of the liberal use of marijuana in the Netherlands, specifically in Amsterdam, between 1986 and 1994. In terms of substance abuse use patterns, the results show that (1) nearly 10 percent of the study population used the substance at least once during the past year; (2) 6 percent used marijuana during the last month; (3) 3 percent of the youth ages 12–15 used the substance, and this rate was rather stable from year to year; (4) among the 20–24-year-olds, which is the age group that reflects the highest pattern of use, "ever use" increased slowly over the time period studied from just under 40 percent in 1987 to 50 percent in 1994, meaning that by the time young people in Amsterdam reached 24 years of age, half of them had smoked a joint or pipe on at least one occasion; (5) in terms of last-month use, the picture over the years is again very stable. Roughly 1 out of every 6 (residents of Amsterdam) in the 20–24-year age group, the group with the most active nightlife in the city, smoked a joint or more; (6) among people older than 24 years, the rate of monthly marijuana use tends to drop off. In Amsterdam, people over the 25–35-year age group show less enthusiasm for the substance, and those in their 50s lose interest almost altogether. Based on the information collected, it can be said with confidence that marijuana use, in contrast to alcohol use, is strongly bound to a phase of life. When used, it is chiefly something for the 16–35-year age group; (7) throughout the years of the study, about 20 to 25 percent of those who use marijuana do so on a continuous basis, and 65 percent of this group use the substance at most twice per week. Smoking the substance more than 20 times a month was infrequent—only 4 percent of those who use it continuously. In comparison, 13 percent of those who use alcohol on a continuous basis drink more than 20 times a month; (8) the average age of first marijuana use is not around 15 but 20, and the median age is 18; (9) the number of new marijuana users per year is very stable, about 1 percent of the population of 12 years or older; and, from the data (years 1990 and 1994), about 10 percent of all marijuana users quit each year and the average age of those people who stop marijuana use is 26; (10) the increase in marijuana availability in Amsterdam has not led to any intensification of use patterns; and (11) lifetime (marijuana) use in Amsterdam, in a climate of total decriminalization, is no higher than in the United States, where use of the substance is associated with a degree of criminalization.

In his study, Cohen addresses the important issue of marijuana as a stepping-stone to other drugs. According to the data collected, a portion of the marijuana users in Amsterdam has had experience with other drugs. But three-quarters to two-thirds (dependent on the age group) of those who ever used marijuana never used any other illegal drug. In other words, in Amsterdam's population there is a group of people who want to experience illegal drugs, but for the majority of these people marijuana use is sufficient. Furthermore, based on available data, marijuana users who take additional drugs are small in number and do so only very infrequently. In the Amsterdam population, "there is little evidence to support the stepping stone or gateway theory."[51]

In sum, it can be said that after more than 20 years of liberal policy toward the use of marijuana, two important observations can be made: (1) in the Netherlands the prevalence of marijuana use does not appear to be any higher than what exists in other countries where the use is still aggressively prosecuted and punished.[52] The prevalence of marijuana use in the Netherlands even seems to decline, in spite of the absence of any form of public pressure or policies targeted against it; and (2) apparently marijuana has found its place in the Dutch variety of socially integrated drugs. "It can be assumed that rules and techniques have been generated in relatively easy going atmospheres that help regulate and control use."[53]

NOTES

1. Grinspoon, L., and Bakalar, J. (1993). *Marijuana: The Forbidden Medicine*. New Haven, CT: Yale University Press (and the Lindesmith Center), p. 1.

2. Ibid., p. 2.

3. Snyder, S. (1970). What have we forgotten about pot. *New York Times Magazine*, December 13, pp. 27, 121, 124, 130; Ray, O., and Ksir, C. (1990) *Drugs, Society and Human Behavior*. St. Louis, MO: Times Mirror/Mosby, p. 325.

4. Baudelaire, C. (1971). *Artificial Paradises; on Hashish and Wine as Means of* Expanding Individuality. Trans. E. Fox. New York: Herder and Herder; Ray and Ksir, p. 327.

5. Makuriya, T. (ed.) (1973). *Marijuana: Medical Papers, 1839–1972*. Oakland, CA: MediComp; Grinspoon and Bakalar, pp. 2–3.

6. Nahas, G. (1975). *Marijuana—Deceptive Weed*. New York: Raven Press; Mann, P. (1985). *Marijuana Alert*. New York: McGraw-Hill; Goode, E. (1989). *Drugs in American Society*. New York: McGraw-Hill, p. 145.

7. Goode, p. 145.

8. Schlosser, E. (1994). Reefer madness. *The Atlantic Monthly*, August, p. 48.

9. Ray and Ksir, p. 327.

10. Snyder, p. 130; Ray and Ksir, p. 327.

11. Schlosser, p. 49.

12. Ibid.

13. Ray and Ksir, p. 328.

14. Grinspoon and Bakalar, p. 4.

15. Ray and Ksir, p. 328.

16. Grinspoon and Bakalar, p. 4.

17. Whitlock, L. (1970). Review: marijuana. *Crime and Delinquency Literature* 2, no. 3: 367; Ray and Ksir, p. 328.

18. Ray and Ksir, p. 328–329.

19. Ibid., p. 329.

20. Ibid.

21. Solomon, D. (ed.) (1966). *Mayor LaGuardia's Committee on Marijuana: The Marijuana Papers*. New York: New American Library; Ray and Ksir, p. 330.

22. Ray and Ksir, p. 330.

23. Eastland, J. (1974). *Marijuana-Hashish Epidemic and Its Impact on United States Security*. Washington, DC: U.S. Government Printing Office.

24. Ibid., p. xv.

25. Goode, p. 150.

26. Sussman, S., Stacy, A., Dent, C., Simon, T., and Johnson, C. (1996). Marijuana use: Current issues and new research directions. *Journal of Drug Issues* 26, no. 4: 700–702.

27. Pollan, M. (1997). Living with medical marijuana. *New York Times Magazine*, July 20, p. 23.

28. Soros, G. (1997). *It's Time to Just Say No to Self-destructive Prohibition*. New York: Lindesmith Center.

29. Pollan, p. 40.

30. Cohen, P. (1990). *Cocaine and Cannabis: an Identical Policy for Different Groups*. Amsterdam: Center of Drug Research, University of Amsterdam, p. 5.

31. Ibid., p. 6.

32. Ray and Ksir, pp. 328–329.

33. Gusfield, J. (1967). *Symbolic Crusade: Status Politics and the American Temperance Movement*. Urbana: University of Illinois Press; Goode, p. 122.

34. Rhodes, W., Hyatt, R., and Scheiman, P. (1994). The price of cocaine, heroin and marijuana, 1981–1993. *Journal of Drug Issues* 24, no. 3: 394–395.

35. Grinspoon and Bakalar, p. 5.

36. U.S. Congress, House Ways and Means Committee, Hearings on H.R. 6385:Taxation of Marijuana, 75th Congress, 1st session, April 27, 1937, 91–94.

37. Grinspoon and Bakalar, p. 5.

38. Peele, S. (1995). Assumptions about drugs and the marketing of drug policies. In W. Bickel and R. DeGrandpre (eds.), *Drug Policy and Human Nature*. New York: Plenum and the Lindesmith Center, p. 1.

39. Schlosser, E. (1997). More reefer madness. *The Atlantic Monthly*, April, pp. 90–102.

40. Glass, S. (1997). Don't you D.A.R.E. *The New Republic*, March 3, pp. 18–28.

41. Johnston, L., O'Malley, P., and Bachman, J. (1987). Psychotherapeutic, licit, and illicit use of drugs among adolescents. *Journal of Adolescent Health* 8: 41.

42. Willard, J., and Schoenborn, C. (1995). Relationship between cigarette smoking and other unhealthy behaviors among our nation's youth: United States, 1992. *Advance Data* 263, April 24. Washington, DC: National Center for Health Statistics, p. 4.

43. Schlosser, p. 90.

44. Wren, C. (1996). Marijuana use by youths continues to rise. *New York Times*, February 20, p. A11.

45. Gfroerer, J., Greenblatt, J., and Wright, D. (1997) Substance use in the US college-age population: Differences according to educational status and living arrangement. *American Journal of Public Health* 87, no. 1: 63.

46. Henneberger, M. (1994). "Pot" surges back, but it's, like, a whole new world. *New York Times*, (IE), February 6, p. 4.

47. National Institute on Drug Abuse (NIDA). (1996). *Epidemiologic Trends in Drug Abuse*. Vol. 1, *Highlights and Executive Summary*. Rockville, MD: National Institutes of Health.

48.de Kort, M. (1994). The Dutch cannabis debate, 1968–1976. *Journal of Drug Issues*: 417–418.

49. Ibid.; Cohen, P. (1988). The Dutch experience: The place of Dutch drug policy in a general framework of social administration. Paper presented at the International CORA Conference on Anti-Prohibition, September 29, October 1.

50. Cohen, P. (1995). Cannabis users in Amsterdam. Paper presented at the National Conference on the Urban Softdrugs Tolerance Policy, Utrecht, June 7, pp. 2–3.

51. Ibid., p. 7.

52. Sijlbing, G. (1984). Introduction, *Het gebruik van drugs, alcohol en tabak*. Amsterdam: Swoad.

53. Cohen, P. (1990). *Cocaine and cannabis: an identical policy for different drugs*. Amsterdam: Centrum voor Drugsonderzoek, pp. 7–8.

Chapter 7

Management: Elements of Drug Treatment Services Organization and Development

HUMAN SERVICES PERSPECTIVE

Inevitably, every person conducts voluntarily or involuntarily transactions with a range of organizations whose explicit purpose is to shape, change, and control behavior as well as confirm or redefine social and personal status. The primary function of human services organizations is to enhance the well-being of a person through functions that are conducted on two levels—societal and individual.[1] Within this context, human services organizations have three major functions. First, these organizations assume major responsibilities for the socialization of people into various roles they may occupy. Second, human service organizations serve as major social control agents by identifying individuals who fail to conform to their role prescriptions and by removing them, at least temporarily, from these role positions. Third, these organizations assume a social integration function by providing the means and resources for individuals to become integrated in the various social units with which they affiliate. Through such mechanisms as resocialization, therapy, counseling, and so on, human service organizations attempt to prevent social disintegration and promote the integration of the individual to society.[2]

A significant body of theoretical knowledge and empirical research exists regarding the organization and management of human services.[3] In this context, theoretical approaches and tools such as operations research and management information systems have much to contribute to understanding and improving the provision of services[4]; however, they tend to be based on assumptions that often cannot be met. Even the fundamental organization development procedure of needs assessment and planning that includes such basic tasks as: (1) information gathering and problem definition; (2) setting objectives (or describing options) and prioritizing them; (3) choosing objectives (or options) and allocating resources; and (4) collecting data on program or service implementation and then interpreting the information to improve services provision is many times ignored.[5]

DRUG TREATMENT SERVICES

Human service organizations tend to provide a predominant type of service to a particular class of clients. For drug treatment organizations, the goal is to improve the well-being of addicts who are perceived to be malfunctioning. In this sense, these organizations may be characterized as people-changing mechanisms. They attempt to alter the attributes or behavior of their clients through various modification and treatment technologies.[6]

For the most part, drug addicts have identifiable social locations and social affiliations that cannot be ignored by the service organization. The social background of drug addicts serves as a critical indicator of the type of treatment services required, their potential for change, and the desired outcomes. Also, affiliation and reference social groups (including family and peers) of the addict have considerable influence on that person's motivation and behavioral patterns that need be considered by the organization in order to maximize the effectiveness of its interventions and to minimize the potential conflict between the services it provides and the ascribed affiliations and social status of the addict.

Drug service organizations define their goals in relation to given tasks such as the detoxification of addicts, secondary and tertiary prevention activities and so on[7]; and, within such a task environment, the organizations are often faced with addressing multiple, often conflicting expectations and interests in terms of results. For example, in attempting to define goals, drug service organizations encounter diverse interest groups that influence their domains and mandates. Among these are (1) the police, concerned with the punishment and removal of the addicts from the community, especially since drug users are known to be the cause of much criminal activity. Regarding this point, the National Institute of Justice, for example, estimates up to 80 percent of offenders, parolees, and probationers have some degree of substance abuse problem related to their criminal activity; more than half of the inmates in local jails report being under the influence of drugs or alcohol at the time of their offense[8]; (2) welfare departments, responsible for a range of social and related support services to families affected by the problem behavior and dysfunction of addicts; (3) local and regional government agencies, responsible for controlling and ameliorating the drug problem; (4) legislators, who see the police, courts, service agencies, and schools as the means to implement social control over drug use; and (5) parents, wives, children, and significant others, who rely on drug service organizations to resolve conflicts and address the needs of the addicts and their families. Often these diverse interest groups are in competition and conflict over defined responsibilities and limited resources that tend to weaken their ability or desire to communicate and coordinate services.

Another factor affecting service provision may be dissonance among staff. Professional and paraprofessional personnel, differentiated by their organization location and work status, including factors such as academic background and personal experience with drugs, may have different ideologies of providing treatment and services to their clients. The greater the occupational, professional, and personal diversity in the drug service organization, the greater the difficulties in developing an internal consensus toward the goals of prevention and treatment of drug use, the control and supervision of staff, minimizing interpersonal conflict, and maintaining cooperation and coordination of efforts.[9]

Considerable energy and resources have been invested in controlling and preventing "war" efforts against drug use. In contrast, relatively little attention appears to have been given to the need for well-organized and managed drug treatment services, including aftercare relapse prevention. Inclusive of this last point are issues of professional and paraprofessional manpower development through skills enhancement, career education, and in-service training opportunities; methods of consultation and technical assistance; supervision of management and direct service personnel; uniformity of information and data collection across locations and over time; and improved methods of needs assessment, evaluation, and research of the long-term effects of service provision including aftercare for the addict and the family.

MANAGEMENT OF DRUG SERVICES

Management

The word "management" implies a very active and constructive development approach that involves the generation, utilization, and possibly reshaping of resources. It is considered an organization-related function that must be (1) concerned with the biopsychosocial distresses faced by addicts and their families and (2) responsive to those arrangements that must be made to address and, hopefully, relieve any or all of the distresses being experienced. Central to this approach is an emphasis on the following principles: (1) drug-related distress, including the relapse or return to a drug-using state after detoxification, may be founded in social system deficiencies rather than physiological, metabolic, genetic, or intrapsychic disorders. Rather than focusing on diagnostic labels that obscure these social system elements, increased concern should be given to the daily "problems of living" adversely affecting addicts and their families; (2) the drug-related prevention and treatment activities given by caregivers have many qualities in common. Competence is the critical variable, and it transcends arbitrary distinctions of academic degree, discipline, and role status (e.g., manager/direct service provider or professional/paraprofessional) in the service provision process; (3) accessibility of drug treatment and prevention services often is as important as their quality to clients seeking appropriate help. Accessibility must be viewed in terms of convenience (e.g., location and appropriate hours of service provision to permit clients to work) as well as psychological comfort (to the addict) involving competent and humanistically oriented staff; (4) systems of service properly integrated to ensure continuity of care are more effective than single services functioning in isolation. The range of human problems associated with drug addiction is so broad that only in exceptional instances can a given organization/agency or unit fully meet the total needs of an addict. There is a tendency among many drug services to reflect a "heap of parts" rather than an integrated network of activities working together; and (5) drug service providers are accountable to multiple constituencies, including clients. Determinations of program effectiveness must include the perspectives of the addicts and their families as well as those of the clinicians, administrators, and resource providers.[10]

The word "management" implies more than being responsive to a central authority and loyal to established policies. It should include actions that are development-oriented, reflect the assertion of leadership, and demonstrate a certain amount of risk taking if service provision is to improve. The idea of drug services management is a bidirectional dilemma that reflects issues of incremental improvements versus substantial reform. Are these two approaches congruent? There are many instances when certain actions can be taken immediately, within an existing structure, to improve the management of drug services. Such efforts (e.g., new and innovative activities to prevent the addict from relapse; in-service technical assistance to improve service provision; staff, volunteer, and paraprofessional training; and community leadership development training to combat drug use), however, must be planned as part of a larger, long-range strategy of service provision reform.[11]

Assessment of Drug Treatment Services Organization and Management

At every level (national, regional, and local) and type of drug service provision (e.g., prevention and treatment), there should be a reasonably accurate assessment of needs of the client. Also, this is true for the service provider, particularly where knowledgeable and experienced personnel, working with adequate resources, are in short supply. Long-range organization development is absolutely dependent on knowing the nature and scope of such needs. Because such needs change over time as a result of new policies and decisions, economic conditions, shifting population trends, and so on, such information gathering or needs assessment should be current.[12]

The assessment of drug treatment services provision is a complicated process because of the multiple dimensions that must be taken into account, such as management needs and problems, organization development obstacles, manpower development and training, research, and so on. In the remaining portion of this chapter, the results of a drug services organization and management assessment, conducted in an exploratory manner, are discussed.

Drug Service Agencies: Organization and Management Needs and Problems

The system of service delivery for drug abuse treatment comprises various private and public service organizations, including specialty treatment, physical and mental health care, social service, correctional, and self-help organizations. Though there has been some progress in the study of organizations that serve drug-abusing patients, treatment organizations remain one of the least studied areas in drug abuse health services research. Given the profound changes that these organizations are currently experiencing, there is a critical need for knowledge on how best to structure and manage service delivery to ensure positive patient outcomes. This information must, however, build upon proven organizational and management research findings across multiple disciplines.[13]

In order to provide policy and program decision makers with a better understanding of the organization and management needs of drug services, a study was made of 12 drug treatment agencies located in a region with a population of 350,000.[14] The directors and managers of these agencies reported that services were being provided to nearly 600 addicts, or 17 percent of the estimated 3,500 drug addicts of the area.

The self-report questionnaires used to collect data for the investigation were developed from major studies of human services organizations.[15] (Appendix B provides an outline of the issues and questions used for the study.) It is common to question whether honest results can be expected from any self-report questionnaire, including the data collection instruments used for this effort, when it involves issues of a sensitive nature such as personal attitudes and behavior. This issue has come under increasing scrutiny, and while concerns are expressed about the adequacy of available measures,[16] the preponderance of studies, including the one presented in this chapter, show that self-report measures of sensitive issues stand up well to tests of reliability and validity.[17]

Drug Service Agencies, Personnel, and Clients: A Description of the Findings

Among the drug service agencies surveyed, six to eight months was the common length of time for treatment provided to addicts. Half of the agencies reported providing some follow-up services to the addicts after their treatment; however, the majority (80 percent) reported that they did not work with family members as part of the treatment process. Also, most of the treatment agencies reported that their efforts were coordinated with other services and that only 24 addicts were waiting for treatment.

Approximately 73 percent (41) of the 56 paid staff providing drug treatment had professional status with an academic degree primarily in social work. Among the 27 percent (15) paraprofessional staff, the majority were former addicts. Volunteers (17) accounted for an additional element of the drug services workforce. Based on the number of professional, paraprofessional, and volunteer personnel involved with the treatment process, the ratio of full-time staff to drug addicts was 1:10. In spite of this, 60 percent of the agency management personnel reported that they had too many drug addicts to serve and not enough staff. Regarding work responsibilities, the majority of staff (62 percent) provided direct support service to the addicts;

21 percent were engaged in administrative and management-related tasks; and 17 percent reported that they were primarily responsible for in-service training. The ratio of management to direct service staff was 1:3.

A significant finding of this study was that not more than 20 percent of the addicts in the target area were accounted for in treatment, follow-up care services, or participation with drug addiction anonymous groups. Also, it was found that 75 percent of the male and 87 percent of the female addicts receiving treatment had problems with alcohol. About 10 percent of those receiving treatment were women, and another 10 percent were youth under the age of 18.

Services and Manpower Development

Drug services in the region reflected a loosely bound network of agencies and units focused on short-term treatment provision. Among the major problems reported by agency personnel were that direct service workers and supervisors had difficulty identifying cases and clients that needed attention; professional staff were performing functions that could be handled by lower-level staff or volunteers; and case records tended to be unorganized and inaccurate. Areas of development assistance reported by agency directors, managers, and drug counselors included the need to improve counseling and treatment skills of direct service workers, the ability to provide treatment to an increased number of addicts, and treatment planning for individuals.

Training

Training was examined from three perspectives: organization, incentives, and priorities. Among the organization issues were the need for drug agencies to provide staff with adequate financial assistance and time off from work in order to be trained; the need for better coordination, especially in terms of linking training to the actual practice problems of caseworkers; and the need for assessment to identify the most important issues to be addressed through training. Reasons provided for drug service agency personnel to participate with in-service training included the need to improve professional status and job performance as well as to obtain a license or certificate. Among the training issues that received priority status were individual counseling, interpersonal communications, preventive outreach to clients and families at risk, working with families as part of a total treatment plan, and group counseling. Both management and direct service personnel believed the provision of individual and group treatment should be the priority for training.

In terms of applied research and evaluation activity related to services development, the following issues were identified as important: client needs (e.g., improving treatment intervention strategies, including follow-up services after detoxification); the needs of female partners and the families of addicts; and cost-effective methods of providing drug treatment and support services.

Steps toward Drug Services Management and Development

Drawing from the results of the study, five major areas were identified for attention and discussion: (1) drug services management and managing services with scarce resources, (2) education and training, (3) out reach to critical target populations, (4) treatment and relapse prevention strategies, and (5) research and evaluation.

Drug Services Development and Managing Services with Scarce Resources

Is the existing infrastructure of services and drug treatment personnel capable of doing more? The answer appears to be no, not without the infusion of funding resources to build up the capability of agencies to treat additional addicts. This includes increasing the number of trained treatment and prevention service personnel. It should be noted, however, that simply expanding the services structure is no guarantee that the 80 percent of addicts not connected with drug treatment and prevention services will be motivated to come forward to receive assistance. Responsibility for drug service agency personnel manpower development is likely to fall on the shoulders of the social work profession, including the regional university's department of social work.

Treatment agency staff appear able, albeit with some difficulty, to handle their present client caseloads. In certain locations throughout the region, caring staff do what they can with what resources are available; however, without additional staff positions, a condition of doing more with less in terms of service provision will result in doing less with less. Clearly, a few agencies (certainly not all) appear to be worthy of investment, monitoring and evaluation in order to create "model treatment service centers" for replication and dissemination of "know-how" information throughout the region and country.

Professional women and a model treatment program are needed to address the needs of females addicted to illegal drugs and alcohol. Such a program should seek out female addicts and promote their willingness to undertake treatment. Also, specially trained personnel are needed to address the needs of young addicts under the age of 18. A special treatment unit capable of organizing, coordinating, and/or providing a range of services, including remedial education and vocational training, should be prioritized for both women and youth.

Considerable attention has been generated by the drug problem in terms of its relation to crime and the spread of AIDS. The amount of funding support and effort needed for developing comprehensive treatment approaches, including relapse prevention, education, and vocational opportunities for the addict, community-based activities to strengthen the family as a treatment milieu, the creation of a job bank, and incentives for ex-addicts to work is considerable.

Practically speaking, the population of addicts who seek treatment and who are determined to stay "clean" tends to be a small percentage of those who use illicit drugs on a regular, habitual basis. An even smaller group succeed in stopping their use of drugs. To talk about increasing the number of addicts for treatment services appears to be unrealistic unless strategies are implemented to increase the probability of success. One possible way to achieve this may be the creation of a network of small, community-based clinics or storefronts responsible for (1) the distribution of methadone, (2) support counseling, and (3) information and referral assistance to larger service facilities staffed with personnel experienced in such support services as relapse prevention, vocational training, job placement, family counseling, and so on.

Education and Training

The study findings show that drug service agencies need assistance, training, and education to (1) further develop the capacity to plan and provide treatment and prevention services, (2) improve staff supervision, (3) better manage case records, and (4) promote communications among professional and paraprofessional personnel. A relatively stable workforce of professional and paraprofessional drug service caseworkers and counselors, measured in terms of turnover and years of experience, provides treatment and other services to the addicts. A number of reasons may account for this; for example, the majority of staff are male, who are less likely to follow a wife to another location for change of career purposes; staff tend to be affiliated and loyal to addressing the drug problem; and there is a limited range of mobility within drug treatment and prevention services enabling movement from job to job.

The sense of workforce stability found to exist among the agencies studied is considered a positive element of the drug services organization, justifying an increased investment in training and education opportunities that will improve personnel work skills as well as promote career opportunities within drug services. Incentives, including time off from the job to pursue training and education, certification, promotion, salary increases, and a university degree, are important to motivate personnel and promote their development as well attract new professionals and paraprofessionals to drug services prevention and treatment. In terms of university education, such opportunities should be based on a flexible model of professional education that includes mechanisms for self-paced study, independent study, concentrated study, small-group and seminar-tutorial methods, project or problem-centered study, practicum or clinical experience, and work-study programs, off-campus study, and internships.[18] These mechanisms should link professional and paraprofessional staff to education and training opportunities as much as possible; however, there should be opportunities to address the unique characteristics of these two work/responsibility distinctions. Also, agency staff should be linked to university social work students as well as other academic/clinical training departments (e.g., medicine, nursing, occupational therapy, recreation, education) to enhance intergroup learning among those involved or those who will be involved with drug services provision.

An additional thought regarding drug training and education is the need for a "new careers movement" to respond to the limited availability of professionals and the high cost of their services. Less formally trained individuals of a paraprofessional nature should be developed to address drug prevention and treatment service needs, including outreach to addicts and their families in the community. Experimental and program research has shown that paraprofessionals may be quite successful in the delivery of specific services, particularly when they are under professional supervision. This suggests that there is a degree of generality in helping behavior. An individual who shows characteristics such as empathy, sensitivity, and a positive regard for others is likely to be an effective helper. Many community people with little or no formal training may be effective helpers.[19]

The trend toward the use of paraprofessionals has contributed to the belief that responsibility should depend on competence in the job to be done rather than on formal training in a particular professional discipline. In addition, the development of nontraditional community resources to deal with drug dependency and the general growth of self-help groups in other community problem areas have created doubt about the value of traditional professional jurisdictional privileges.[20]

Although paraprofessionals lack formal training and the specific degrees of professionals, they have demonstrated competence as drug service workers on the basis of practical experience and generalist training.[21] With this in mind, a paraprofessional drug specialist training program may prove to be a very worthwhile investment for manpower development purposes. Such a program should be tied to career development opportunities, including access to an education and training program with elements of community work, individual and family counseling, drug treatment and prevention, therapeutic recreation, job counseling and placement, occupational therapy, special education, and self-help services organization (e.g., Narcotics Anonymous).

In addition to trained and educated professional and paraprofessional staff, the success of local drug treatment service provision, including community-based methadone maintenance clinics, may be dependent, in part, on the extent that community leaders can be developed. Leadership at the local level capable of addressing the problem of drug use would seem to have two preconditions: (1) a person who has conceptual skills and good interpersonal relations and (2) an environment responsive to, and perhaps even needing, change.

Outreach: Critical Target Populations

The study findings reveal that special outreach and treatment services are needed for three client populations including (1) the 80 percent or more of the drug addict population that appears to have no contact with drug service agencies for treatment, aftercare, or other forms of intervention services; (2) female addicts; and (3) adolescent drug users.

Drug Addicts in Need of Services. Outreach efforts that encourage addicts to participate in a treatment program and the ability to provide successful treatment may both be grounded in the provision of services that relate to relapse prevention, education and vocational training, support of the family as part of the treatment milieu, work, community-based social and recreational activities, and suitable housing.

Generally speaking, the vast majority of drug addicts do not receive treatment services; therefore, 80 percent or more of this group may be targets for outreach activity that involve workers knowledgeable about the drug problem, skilled in talking to people, and capable of promoting motivation in order to turn their lives around. One of the important reasons for drug outreach service is to provide information, since many addicts are unaware of their rights for treatment, the types of assistance available, and how to access help. For example, the outreach worker might make an appointment for a person at a community agency and he may talk to the agency in behalf of the addict and help set the stage for his entry into a treatment program. Also, the drug outreach worker may have an important role in helping the addict feel more at ease in using community services, since there is a tendency to be afraid or reluctant to talk about lifestyle, especially since it is likely to involve illegal drug use, crime, abuse, violence, and prostitution. Finally, the outreach worker can assist the community in learning about the people in need of drug service, particularly those who have not come to the attention of others.[22] While many details need to be considered and developed further, especially in terms of the specific tasks to be undertaken by the outreach worker, the need to recruit ex-addicts, including women, who are familiar with the community for this role is important.

Female Drug Addicts. The results of this study reveal that only 9–10 percent of the addicts receiving treatment are women, when it is believed that as much as 20 percent of the addicted population is female. Clearly, additional research is needed to understand why this percentage is so low. Among the possible explanations is that women may be more able than men to sustain their addiction to drugs through illegal income-earning activities such as prostitution, and/or their partners may be providing drugs or supplying the money necessary to purchase drugs. In either situation, there may be little need or interest to seek sources of support for their addiction or incentive to go through processes of detoxification and treatment. Regarding treatment, there tends to be a lack of gender-specific services, including individual and group counseling for female addicts. The world of drug addiction treatment appears to be a male domain; consequently, female addicts may feel (and rightly so) out of place in a treatment facility and becoming involved with the services provided if they are not gender-specific.

In a study by the U.S. National Institute of Drug Abuse (NIDA) it has been found that at the end of 1994, 58,000 women were reported to be HIV-infected and 41 percent of these cases resulted from injection drug use. Indeed, women's drug and sex risks for HIV frequently occur together. Women's drug use often involves membership in a network with HIV-infected individuals where direct and indirect sharing of injection equipment and/or sexual liaisons are transacted and where the social context (e.g., shooting gallery) affects the likelihood of transmitting HIV. According to NIDA, drug-dependent women are more likely than men to engage in high-risk sex, and women who inject drugs are more likely to acquire HIV sexually than men. Violence may be an additional risk factor. This is because women with abusive partners practice more HIV-risk behaviors and are less likely to seek drug treatment or disclose their HIV status to their partners than nonabused women. Women's unique HIV transmission context and behaviors, including the link between drug dependence and risky sex as well as the potential transmission to infants, have implications for the development of targeted, gender-specific, risk-related interventions.[23]

While the proportion of HIV and female drug users is expected to vary from city to city and nation to nation, it is an issue that must be considered one of the most serious drug-related problems. Outreach activities targeted to female drug users and gender-specific treatment programs, including individual and group counseling as well as relapse prevention activities, must be given priority development status.

Adolescent Drug Users. According to Brown and Mills

[w]ork in the field of prevention programming has emphasized the development of large-scale efforts designed to contain drug use throughout the adolescent population. Given the pernicious character of drug abuse, and its endemic nature in this country, it is not surprising that there has been an emphasis on providing educational experiences and prevention programs for a general adolescent population. But at the same time, it has been increasingly recognized that certain elements of the adolescent population are distinctly more at risk for substance abuse than others. Most notably, those living in communities in which there is widespread availability of illicit substances, and whose experiences more largely distance them from the larger society, can be viewed as at greater risk for substance abuse.[24]

Among the populations of young people who may be considered at high risk are delinquent youth, children of substance abusers, runaways, school dropouts, and those placed outside the home of their "natural parents" in foster care or an institutional setting. Using the children of substance abusers as an example, psychosocial studies have found that the offspring of alcoholics often exhibit cognitive and interpersonal problems as children and general psychiatric disturbances and alcoholism as adults. Also, it has been shown that parental and sibling illicit drug use increases the youth's risk of alcoholism and drug abuse.[25] The majority of clients in treatment for alcohol and drug abuse have had chemically dependent parents or relatives.[26]

Clearly, high-risk youth need special attention to prevent and if necessary, treat their addiction to alcohol and/or drugs.

Strategies must be developed for identifying those youngsters in need of drug abuse services and for coordinating the work of agencies treating substance abuse and other dysfunctional behaviors. Interventions may make use of existing staff at the community agencies treating the presenting problem or may involve referral to drug abuse treatment programs. In either case, innovative [programs] using skills training and/or other psycho-social strategies will need to be developed and evaluated, and agency staff will need to receive the training necessary [that contributes to the identification of drug abusers and promotes response(s) appropriate to their needs].[27]

TREATMENT AND RELAPSE PREVENTION STRATEGIES

A range of intervention strategies has been discussed. What has been said and should be said again is that the treatment of drug addicts must go beyond detoxification and reaching-out activities. A program of relapse prevention, including family social and recreational services as well as work opportunities (e.g., public facility repair jobs that offer a small financial incentive for a few hours of work each day in addition to welfare payments), should be made available as part of a "total" treatment program.

In providing support to addicts, it must be realized this is not a homogeneous group. In other words, each addict has his or her unique personality and physical characteristics. Too often in the provision of human services, there is a tendency to provide clients with only the services that are available. If a client does not match the service(s), there is a good chance that the individual will fall through the cracks between programs and not receive the service(s) needed. Attention must be given to those addicts who are unique because of their physical (i.e., the handicapped or disabled) or mental (i.e., mentally retarded or mentally ill) characteristics. Appropriate diagnosis, planning, intervention, and follow-up are vital to address the needs of these difficult subgroups within a difficult population.

RESEARCH AND EVALUATION

From the study conducted, numerous subjects for additional research were identified. These include high-risk populations in terms of abusing drugs, such as (1) the children of addicts, runaways, youth who drop out of school, as well as patterns and problems of child and spouse abuse caused by alcoholics and drug addicts; (2) the needs of the female addicts, issues regarding drug use and prostitution among women, patterns of child care when the mother is addicted; issues of codependence involving the wife or female partner of the addict and her role in the addiction process as well as treatment and relapse prevention; and (3) the population of addicts who do not pursue treatment compared to those who are involved with treatment and aftercare services such as Narcotics Anonymous.

Additional research and evaluation efforts may include the validation of programs and services "that work," evaluation of technical assistance and training to agency staff, job satisfaction among professional and paraprofessional workers, job burnout, the work values orientation among addicts in various stages of the recovery process, and the patterns of recidivism and success among addicts and their families who have been affected by illegal drug and alcohol use.

NOTES

1. Hasenfeld, Y., and English, R. (1978). *Human Service Organizations*. Ann Arbor: University of Michigan Press, pp. 1–2.

2. Ibid.; Likert, R. (1967). *The Human Organization*. New York: McGraw-Hill; Moos, R. (1975). *Evaluating Correctional and Community Settings*. New York: John Wiley and Sons; Patti, R., Poertner, J., and Rapp, C. (eds.) (1988). *Managing for Services Effectiveness in Social Welfare Organizations*. New York: Haworth Press.

3. Hasenfeld, Y. (ed.) (1992). *Human Services As Complex Organizations*. Newbury Park, CA: Sage Publications; Hasenfeld and English; Sarri, R., and Hasenfeld, Y. (1978). *The Management of Human Services*. New York: Columbia University Press; Robbins, S. (1987). *Organization Theory: Structure, Design, and Applications*. Englewood Cliffs, NJ: Prentice-Hall International Editions; Burke, A., and Clapp, J. (1997). Ideology and social work practice in substance abuse settings. *Social Work* 42, no. 6: 553.

4. Hasenfeld and English, p. 22

5. Delahanty, D. (1980). *The Comprehensive Plan: Strategies for Human Services*. Louisville, KY: Human Services Coordination Alliance.

6. Hasenfeld and English, p.6; Hasenfeld.

7. Moos; Patti, R., Poertner, J., and Rapp, C. (eds.) (1988). *Managing for Services Effectiveness in Social Welfare Organizations*. New York: Haworth Press; DuPont, R. (1989). Stopping Alcohol and Other Drug Use Before It Starts: The Future of Prevention. AOSAP Prevention Monograph 1; Rockville, MD: U.S. Department of Health and Human Services, Office of Substance Abuse; Pickens, R., Leukefeld, C., and Schuster, C. (1991). *Improving Drug Abuse Treatment*, Research Monograph 106, Rockville, MD: U.S. Department of Health and Human Services, National Institute on Drug Abuse.

8. Harlow, C. W. (1991). *Drugs and Jail Inmates, 1989*. Bureau of Justice Statistics, Special Report. Washington, DC: U.S.Department of Justice.

9. Hasenfeld and English, p. 7; Baron, R. (1986). *Behavior in Organizations*. Boston: Allyn and Bacon.

10. Demone, H. (1978). *Stimulating Human Services Reform, Human Services Monograph Series*. Project Share. Washington, DC: U.S. Department of Health, Education, and Welfare.

11. Curtis, W. (1981). *Managing Human Services with Less; New Strategies for Local Leaders*. Project Share. Washington, DC: U.S. Department of Health, Education, and Welfare.

12. Delahanty, D. (1978). *The Community Profile*. Louisville, KY: Human Services Coordination Alliance.

13. D'Aunno, T., and Vaughn, T. (1995). The organizational analysis of service patterns in outpatient drug abuse treatment units. *Journal of Substance Abuse* 7: 27–42; D'Aunno, T., and Price, R. (1986). Linked systems: Drug abuse and mental health services. In W. R. Scott and Black, B. L. (eds.), *The Organization of Mental Health Services: Societal and Community Systems*. Beverly Hills, CA: Sage Publications; Timko, C. (1995). Policies and services in residential substance abuse programs: Comparisons with psychiatric programs. *Journal of Substance Abuse* 7: 43; National Institute on Drug Abuse (NIDA). (1997). *Organization and Management of Drug Abuse Treatment Services*. NIH Guide, vol. 26, no. 16, May 16.

14. Isralowitz, R., Telias, D., and Tabu, N. (1996). *Drug Services in the Negev: A Study of Organization Problems and Needs, Staff Training and Treatment Issues: A report to the*

Negev Development Authority. Beer Sheva: Department of Social Work, Ben-Gurion University of the Negev.

15. Sundel, M. (1979). *Local Child Welfare Services Self-Assessment Manual, Part 1—Checklists.* Washington, DC: Social Services Research Program, The Urban Institute; Vinokur, D., and Jackson, G. (1981). *Attitudes and Evaluation of In-Service Training by Local Administrators.* Ann Arbor: National Child Welfare Training Center, University of Michigan.

16. Amor, D., Polich, J., and Stambul, H. (1978). Reliability and validity of self-reported drinking behavior. In D. Amor, J. Polich, and H. Stambul (eds.), *Alcoholism and Treatment.* New York: John Wiley and Sons, pp. 173–211; Rouse, B., Kozel, N., and Richards, L. (eds.) (1985). *Self-Report Methods of Estimating Drug Use: Meeting Current Challenges to Validity.* Washington, DC: NIDA.

17. Engs, R. C. (1977). Drinking patterns and drinking problems of college students. *Journal of Studies on Alcohol* 39: 2144–2156; Johnston, L., and O'Malley, P. (1985). Issues of validity and population coverage in student surveys of drug use. In B. Rouse, M. Kozel, and L. Richards (eds.), *Self-Report Methods of Estimating Drug Use: Meeting Current Challenges to Validity.* Washington, DC: NIDA, pp. 31–54; Johnston, L., O'Malley, P., and Bachman, J. (1992). *Smoking, Drinking, and Illicit Drug Use among American Secondary Students, College Students, and Young Adults, 1975–1991,* vols. 1&2. Washington, DC: NIDA; O'Malley, P., Carey, K., and Maisto, S. (1986). Validity of young adults' reports of parental drinking practices. *Journal of Studies on Alcohol* 47: 433–435; Williams, G., Aitken, S., and Malin, H. (1985). Reliability of self-reported alcohol consumption in a general population. *Journal of Studies on Alcohol* 46: 223–227.

18. Burnford, F., and Chenault, J. (1978). *The Current State of Human Services Professional Education.* Project Share. Washington, DC: U.S. Department of Health, Education, and Welfare.

19. Chenault, J., and Burnford, F. (1978). *Human Services Professional Education.* New York: McGraw-Hill; Cowen, E. (1973). Social and community interventions. In P. Mussen and M. Rosenzweig (eds.), *Annual Review of Psychology.* Palo Alto, CA: Annual Reviews; Krebs, D. (1970). Altruism—an examination of the concept and a review of the literature. *Psychological Bulletin* 73: 258–302; Levine, M., and Graziano, A. (1972). Intervention programs in elementary schools. In S. E. Golann and C. Eisdorfer (eds.), *Handbook of Community Mental Health.* New York: Appleton.

20. Chenault and Burnford; Baker, F. (1977). The interface between professional and natural support systems. *Clinical Social Work Journal* 5: 139–148.

21. Iscoe, I. (1971). Professional and subprofessional training in community mental health as an aspect of community psychology. In Division 27 of the American Psychological Association. *Issues In Community Psychology and Preventive Mental Health.* New York: Behavioral Publications; Chenault and Burnford, p. 158.

22. Cushing, M., and Long, N. (1973). *Reaching Out: Information and Referral Services.* Washington, DC: U.S. Department of Health, Education, and Welfare.

23. National Institute on Drug Abuse (NIDA). (1995). *Women's HIV Risk and Protective Behaviors.* NIH Guide, vol. 24, no. 30, August 18.

24. Brown, B., and Mills, A. (1990). *Youth at Risk for Substance Abuse.* Rockville, MD: U.S. Department of Health and Human Services, NIDA, p. vii.

25. Adler, R., and Raphael, B. (1983). Children of alcoholics. *Australian and New Zealand Journal of Psychiatry* 17: 3–8; Wilson, C. (1982). The impact of children. In J. Orford and J. Harwin (eds.), *Alcohol and the Family.* London: Croom Helm; Thorne, C.,

and DeBlassie, K. (1985). Adolescent substance abuse. *Adolescence* 20, no. 78: 335–347; Kumpfer, K. (1986). *Prevention Strategies for Children of Drug-Abusing Parents.* Proceedings of the 34th Annual International Congress on Alcoholism and Drug Dependence, Calgary, Alberta.

26. Isralowitz, R., and Singer, M. (eds.) (1983). *Adolescent Substance Abuse: A Guide to Prevention and Treatment.* New York: Haworth; Cotton, N. (1979). The familial incidence of alcoholism. *Journal of Studies on Alcohol* 40, no. 1: 89–116; Goodwin, D. (1971). Is alcoholism hereditary? A review and critique. *Archives of General Psychiatry* 25: 545–549.

27. Brown and Mills, p. 181.

Epilogue: The Final Straw—A Response to the War against Drugs

American society has a major drug problem on its hands; the condition is undesirable, and it appears that policies must be changed, and new programs must be instituted.[1] This statement was made nearly a decade ago, and little has changed based on observations and reports regarding patterns of drug use and addicted behavior, criminal acts, emergency hospital visits, and violence. The opinions expressed by anti-drug leaders, a wide range of respected judicial and government officials, social scientists, and commentators on the social order tend to agree that national drug policy and the war on drugs is a "dismal failure,"[2] "monumental error," and "utter futility."[3] Briefly, the most damning evidence reveals that "the drug market in the United States is estimated at $150 billion a year . . . the rate of incarceration is the highest for any Western nation, almost 1 million in jails or prisons at a cost of $20 billion a year. Federal drug cases have trebled in ten years, up 25 per cent in 1993 alone, with marijuana cases up 17 per cent."[4] The annual federal anti-drug budget for law enforcement has grown from roughly $53 million in 1970, to about 10 billion in fiscal year (FY) 1997; since 1970, the United States has invested roughly $77 billion in domestic and foreign drug enforcement—$74 billion since 1981. America now spends some $3 billion a year on its overseas drug wars alone.[5] A fundamental building block for an anti-drug strategy is treatment; yet

in the past decade, funds for treating drug addiction dropped from 25 percent of the federal drug budget—well before the cocaine epidemic created millions of new addicts—to only 14 percent. In the same period, arrests for drug crimes doubled, while violent crime jumped by more than a third. Half of all offenders arrested for homicide or aggravated assault in 1989 were using cocaine or heroin, as were three-quarters of those arrested for burglary or robbery. . . . Addicts today often face waits of six months or longer before they can get help. Treatment is even more scarce in the criminal justice system. The General Accounting Office reported in 1991 that only 364 of the 41,000 federal prison inmates who have drug problems are participating in intensive day treatment. More than three-quarters of all state prison inmates are drug users—at least 500,000 offenders—but only 10 to 20 percent receive any help . . . although addicts maintained on methadone will give up heroin and commit fewer crimes, such treatment is available to less than 20 percent of the nation's heroin addicts.[6]

In spite of these conditions, declarations are made by the director of the White House's Office of National Drug Control Policy, General Barry McCaffrey, that "this is the country that mobilized itself to put a man on the moon in ten years, that built the interstate highway system and that won the [Persian] Gulf war in 30 days. We never fail. . . . Enough is enough,"[7] and Lee Brown, director of the Office of National Drug Control Policy, has said that strategy is in place providing the nation with a "concise, action-oriented approach to drug prevention and drug treatment, law enforcement, local program implementation, and international/interdiction."[8] These remarks provide little solace to those who know that the "high ground" has not been captured in the war against drugs, and who have come realize that the "emperor's drug war has no clothes."[9]

PREVENTION AND TREATMENT

If the Shoe Doesn't Fit, Why Do We Buy and Wear It?

In the war against drugs, a major battlefront involves prevention and treatment. At best, drug use prevention and treatment programs tend to reflect a mixed bag of results. It appears that a number of intervention strategies have demonstrated the ability to reduce or prevent drug use and drug-related crime. "They cover school and community-based education and prevention, various methods of treatment, drug testing and employee-assistance programs in the workplace, organized neighborhood action to drive out dealers, media campaigns and other efforts to change public attitudes and establish norms of conduct that rule out drug use, and grass-roots coalitions."[10] For the most part, however, drug prevention and treatment efforts have been poorly planned and underfunded and tend to evidence a lack of coordinated services for a variety of historical, political, and economic reasons, including those that relate to the social construction of reality and social values discussed in Chapter 1.

Little hard evidence exists documenting the effectiveness of treatment. Almost nothing is known about (1) the effectiveness of the major types of drug treatment, including residential therapeutic communities; inpatient/outpatient chemical dependency treatment; outpatient methadone maintenance programs; and outpatient nonmethadone treatment; (2) the relative effectiveness of different versions of each treatment modality; and (3) the prognosis for different types of drug abusers. Additionally, drug treatment research raises troublesome issues for policymakers; for example, how can treatment work when clinicians claim that success depends on clients' wanting help, and it is known that most clients are forced into treatment, and what happens to drug abusers who never seek treatment? "What can be said with some certainty is that 1) methadone maintenance programs can help clients who are highly motivated to end their drug abuse, and 2) a model program that provides counseling along with methadone has been able to help less well-motivated clients."[11]

From an economic perspective, simple cost facts do not appear to have had much influence on the way treatment policy has been formulated and resources allocated. A California study has shown, for example, that on average every $1 invested in treatment saves $7 in crime and health care costs.[12] The National Association of State Alcohol and Drug Abuse Directors has estimated that the annual cost to incarcerate a drug offender is up to $50,000 per inmate compared to the annual cost of outpatient, drug-free treatment at $2,300, methadone maintenance at $3,000 per patient, and residential, drug-free treatment at $14,000.[13] "Treatment is available for less than 15 percent of the nation's 5.5 million drug abusers, unless they can afford to pay for private programs. Drug treatment within the criminal justice system is even more limited, although at least half of the 1.1 million offenders currently behind bars have serious drug problems,"[14] and federally appropriated funds for treating drug addiction have actually dropped on a budget proportion basis.[15] From the supply-side drug strategy perspective, once again data appear to have had little influence on the formation of policy and intervention strategies. It has been noted

that even success in the [strategy] of significantly reducing overseas supply through force and coercion would fail to meet the larger political objective for which the war is being fought: raising the street price of drugs in the United States enough to reduce drug abuse and addiction. This is because the actual costs of growing and processing illegal drugs abroad are only a minimal part of the street price in the United States. At the point of export, the price of cocaine is still only 3 to 5 percent of the price a U.S. consumer will pay. Even smuggling costs—from Colombia to the United States—account for less than 5 percent of the retail price . . . [and putting the failure more simply] only four Boeing 747 cargo planes or thirteen trailer trucks could supply U.S. cocaine consumption for a year; the annual U.S. demand for heroin could be met by a twenty-square-mile field.[16]

Drug addicts are not a homogeneous group, and, in theory, the needs of each client should be matched,[17] preferably to a service system characterized by rational, flexible, responsive, well-defined, short- and long-term integrated service plans developed on dependable funding sources with ongoing monitoring and evaluation.[18] The fact remains, however, that such approaches are, for the most part, absent in the United States. "Drug abuse treatment has waxed and waned over the past three decades under different administrations, under different funding priorities, and in response to changing patterns of drug use, drug availability, and perceived national threat."[19]

Despite sporadic efforts by national commissions, policy advisory panels, and federal agencies to develop policies and plans to improve treatment—many of which have detailed the same or similar recommendations for what is needed—the development of drug treatment has more often than not been reactive rather than proactive, piecemeal rather than planned, and fragmented rather than integrated. . . . Current policy and practice isolates [*sic*] the drug abuser from the mainstream of health care; legislation and general policy, including funding priorities, have created often insurmountable barriers to treatment for many people with drug problems.[20]

Drug prevention efforts tend to reflect an equally muddled scene of policy and practice. Specifically, the government invests annually hundreds of millions of dollars in an anti-drug program known as DARE (Drug Abuse Resistance Education). In one evaluation of the program it was found that "the level of drug use among kids who had gone through DARE was virtually identical to the level among kids who had not . . . [and based on multiple outcome measures the conclusion was reached that] DARE exposure does not produce any long-term prevention efforts on adolescent drug use rates."[21] In a 1996 study published in Preventive Medicine it was found that any results from DARE were extremely short-lived, and there was no evidence that the prevention program reduces drug use. In 1994, a National Institute of Justice-sponsored study concluded that "while DARE was loved by teachers and participants, it had no effect on drug use." In response to this finding the Justice Department refused to release the peer-reviewed study; however, the *American Journal of Public Health* accepted it for publication.[22]

THE WAR: AND THE DEBATE GOES ON

In February 1996, the National Review stated the position that the time had come to revise the laws on drug trafficking. "[The *National Review*] deplores the [use of drugs] and we urge the stiffest sentences against anyone convicted of selling a drug to a minor. But that said, it is our judgment that the war on drugs has failed, that it is diverting intelligent energy away from how to deal with the problem of addiction, that it is wasting our resources, and that it is encouraging civil, judicial, and penal procedures associated with police states."[23] Based on a symposium of national experts sponsored by the magazine, the primary conclusions were "1) that the famous drug war is not working; 2) that crime and suffering have greatly increased as a result of prohibition; 3) that we have seen, and are countenancing, a creeping attrition of authentic civil liberties; and 4) that the direction in which to head is legalization."[24]

Efforts to reverse drug prohibition face formidable obstacles,[25] such as anti-drug warlords' control over the attitudes and behavior of those involved with all aspects of drug control, prevention, and treatment through the distribution of funding resources and the "bogeyman syndrome"—the need of people to use scapegoats to:

embody their fears and take blame for whatever ails them. . . . Just as anti-Communist propagandists once feared Moscow far beyond its actual influence and appeal, so today anti-drug proselytizers indict marijuana, cocaine, heroin and assorted hallucinogens far beyond their actual psychoactive effects and psychological appeal. Never mind that the vast majority of Americans have expressed . . . little interest in trying [drugs], even if they were legal, and never mind that most of those who tried them have suffered few, if any, ill effects. The evidence of history and of science is drowned out by today's bogeymen. No rhetoric is too harsh, no penalty too severe.[26]

In spite of this situation and the fact that prospects for reevaluation and reform look dim,[27] history shows that the legal and moral status of psychoactive drugs has kept changing. "During the seventeenth century the sale and use of tobacco were punished by death in much of Europe, Russia, China, and Japan. For centuries many of the same Muslim domains that forbade the sale and consumption of alcohol, at the same time, tolerated and even regulated the sale of opium and cannabis."[28]

In the United States change is occurring, especially at the state level, as evidenced by the California and Arizona initiatives toward marijuana use and the state attorney generals' challenge to the tobacco industry for compensation of health costs and reform. A broad-based coalition of respectable special interest groups and grassroots organizations may prove to be the vanguard for moving drug policy and practices to a more rational and pragmatic level for addressing the problem. Certainly, if this expectation does not come to fruition, there is always the issue of economic realities and constraints. "Americans are not keen on paying the rising costs of enforcing laws,"[29] especially when substantial tax revenues can be generated through different methods of control and regulation. The door is open for change in terms of how the problem of drug use is to be addressed; the only question is when and how that change will occur. Getting there will not be easy, and the effort should be taken incrementally. Such gradualism, which should begin with marijuana, would allow for a necessary shift in values so that more socially and economically pragmatic policies can be formulated and enacted.[30] For some, such legislation may be a leap in the dark. Indeed, there will be unpredictable consequences as well as predictable ones. But that does not argue for doing nothing or talking tougher with words that are empty in terms of action and outcomes.

NOTES

1. Goode, E. (1989). *Drugs in American Society*. New York: McGraw-Hill, p. 261.

2. Russell, A. (1992). Making America drug free: A new vision of what works, *Carnegie Quarterly* 37, no. 3: 1.

3. Sweet, R. (1996). The war on drugs is lost. *National Review*, February 12, p. 44.

4. Ibid.

5. Bertram, E., and Sharpe, K. (1996). The unwinnable drug war: What Clausewitz would tell us. *World Policy Journal* (Winter): 44.

6. Falco, M. (1992). *The Making of a Drug-free America: Programs That Work*. New York: Times Books; Russell, pp. 5–6.

7. Kitfield, J. (1996). Four-star general. *National Journal* 4, no. 13: 823.

8. Brown, L. (1995). *National Drug Control Strategy: Executive Summary*. Washington, DC: Office of National Drug Control Policy, p. i.

9. Bertram and Sharpe, p. 50.

10. Falco; Russell, p. 5.

11. Apsler, R. (1994). Is drug abuse treatment effective? *American Enterprise* (March/April): 53.

12. Gerstein, D., Johnson, R., Harwood, H., Fountain, D., Suter, N., and Malloy, K. (1994). *Evaluating recovery services: The California drug and alcohol treatment assessment.* Sacramento: California Department of Alcohol and Drug Programs.

13. National Institute of Justice. (1993). *Drug Use Forecasting: 1992 Annual Report: Drugs and Crime in America's Cities.* Washington, DC: National Institute of Justice, U.S. Department of Justice; Wellisch, J., Prendergast, M., and Anglin, M. (1995). Toward a drug abuse treatment system. *Journal of Drug Issues* 25, no. 4: 760–761.

14. Russell, p. 3.

15. Ibid., p. 5.

16. Ibid., p. 8.

17. Cohen, A. (1986). A psychosocial typology of drug addicts and implications for treatment. *International Journal of the Addictions* 21, no. 2: 147–154.

18. Downes, E., and Shaening, M. (1993). Linking state AOD and justice systems. *Center for Substance Abuse Treatment TIE Communique* (Spring): 8–9; Wellisch, Prendergast, and Anglin, p. 767.

19. Basteman, K. (1992). Federal leadership in building the national drug treatment system. In D. Gerstein and H. Harwood (eds.), *Treating Drug Problems.* Washington, DC: National Academy Press; Haaga, J., and McGlynn, E. (1990). *The Drug Abuse Treatment Systems: Prospects for Reform.* Santa Monica, CA: Drug Policy Research Center, RAND Corporation; Musto, D. (1987). *The American Disease: Origins of Narcotic Control,* 2nd ed. New York: Oxford University Press; Wellisch, Prendergast, and Anglin, p. 765.

20. McAuliffe, W. (1990). Health care policy issues in the drug abuser treatment field. *Journal of Health Politics, Policy and Law* 15, no. 2: 357–385; see also, Schlesinger, M., and Dorwart, R. (1992). Falling between the cracks: Failing national strategies for the treatment of substance abuse. *Daedalus* 121, no. 3): 195–237; Wellisch, Prendergast, and Anglin, p. 770.

21. Glass, S. (1997). Don't you DARE. *The New Republic,* March 3, p. 20.

22. Ibid.

23. Sweet, p. 34.

24. Buckley, W. (1996). 400 readers give their views. *National Review,* July 1, p. 32.

25. Nadelmann, E. (1993). Should we legalize drugs? History answers. *American Heritage* 44, no. 1: 42.

26. Nadelmann, p. 47.

27. Bertram and Sharpe, p. 50.

28. Nadelmann, p. 47.

29. Ibid.

30. Shopping for a drugs policy. (1997). *The Economist,* August 15, p. 30.

University Student Alcohol Use: Attitudes and Behavior Questionnaire Outline

A: BACKGROUND

Sex
(male/female)

Family status
married
married with children
single
divorced
widow(er)

Date of birth

Field of study
social sciences
humanities
technology
medicine
natural sciences
other (specify)

Which degree are you studying for?
B.A.
M.A.
other (specifiy)

Which year of your studies are you in now?

Your country of birth

Father's country of birth

Mother's country of birth

Father's education
  no formal education
  elementary school
  high school
  teacher's college
  university

Mother's education
  no formal education
  elementary school
  high school
  teacher's college
  university

How would you assess your parent's financial situation?
  very good
  good
  average
  bad
  very bad

Did you serve in the army? (yes/no)
  If yes, how many years

Where do you live when studying at the university?
  on campus
  off-campus (private apartment)
  with parents
  other (specify)

Religion
  Jewish
  Muslim
  Christian
  other (specify)

How would you define yourself in religious terms?
  strictly observant of all religious duties
  partially observant of all the religious duties
  observant only of a few of the religious duties

secular—not religious

How would you define your parents in religious terms?
strictly observant of all religious duties
partially observant of all the religious duties
observant only of a few of the religious duties
secular—not religious

B: ALCOHOL ATTITUDES AND BEHAVIOR

Have you used alcoholic beverages in the past? (yes/no)
If yes, which ones? (specify)

IF YOU DRINK (IN THE PRESENT), PLEASE ANSWER THE FOLLOWING QUESTIONS

Beer

How often do you drink beer?
every day
at least once a week, but not every day
at least once a month, but less than once a week
more than once a year, but less than once a month
once a year or less

When you drink beer, how many cans/bottles on average do you drink each time?
more than 6 cans/bottles
5 or 6 cans/bottles
3 or 4 cans/bottles
1 or 2 cans/bottles
less than 1 can/bottle

Wine

How often do you drink wine?
every day
at least once a week, but not every day
at least once a month, but less than once a week
more than once a year, but less than once a month
once a year or less

When you drink wine, how many glasses on average do you drink each time?
more than 6 glasses
5 or 6 glasses
3 or 4 glasses
1 or 2 glasses
less than 1 glass

"Hard" Alcoholic Beverages (Whiskey, Vodka, Gin, Cocktails, etc.)

How often do you drink "hard" alcoholic beverages?
every day
at least once a week, but not every day
at least once a month, but less than once a week
more than once a year, but less than once a month
once a year or less

When you drink "hard" alcoholic beverages, how many glasses on average do you drink each time?
more than 6 glasses
5 or 6 glasses
3 or 4 glasses
1 or 2 glasses
less than 1 glass

Patterns of Alcohol Use

Do you drive after drinking?
always
often
seldom
never

Do you drink while driving?
always
often
seldom
never

Do you drink in the morning?
always
often
seldom
never

Do you drink before class?
always
often
seldom
never

The questions in the following section describe *side effects* of drinking. Listed below are different frequencies. Please respond to each *side effect* with the most appropriate frequency.

1. never experienced
2. experienced at least once in my life but not during the last year
3. not experienced in the last two months, but experienced at least once during the past year
4. experienced at least once in the last two months

Headache, vomiting or nausea the morning after drinking (__)

Criticized about your drinking habits by someone you know (__)

Loss of a job because of your drinking (__)

Trouble with university or dormitory administrators as a result of behavior caused by drinking (__)

The questions in the following section describe different *behavior related to drinking*, or *behavior as a result of drinking*, as reported by other students. Listed above are the different frequencies. Please mark each incident with the appropriate frequency.

Drinking before class (__)

Not going to class after drinking (__)

Not going to class as a result of a "hangover" (headaches and vomiting after drinking) (__)

Getting into a fight as a result of drinking (__)

Damaging property as a result of drinking (__)

Please Answer the Following Additional Questions:

With whom did you have your first drink? (circle one)
   alone
   friends
   parents
   spouse
   brother/sister
   other relatives
   other (specify)

With whom do you drink most? (circle one)
   alone
   friends
   parents
   spouse
   brother/sister
   other relatives
   other (specify)

To what extent is drinking important among your friends? (circle one)

very important
important
not very important
not at all important

With regard to the following issues, to what extent do you feel that your drinking has a beneficial or a damaging effect? (circle the most appropriate answer)

social relations
beneficial effect (5 pt. scale—very much . . . not at all)
damaging effect (5 pt. scale—very much . . . not at all)

family relations
beneficial effect (5 pt. scale—very much . . . not at all)
damaging effect (5 pt. scale—very much . . . not at all)

academic studies
beneficial effect (5 pt. scale—very much . . . not at all)
damaging effect (5 pt. scale—very much . . . not at all)

work
beneficial effect (5 pt. scale—very much . . . not at all)
damaging effect (5 pt. scale—very much . . . not at all)

health
beneficial effect (5 pt. scale—very much . . . not at all)
damaging effect (5 pt. scale—very much . . . not at all)

Would you be interested in knowing more about the effects drinking has on your health and functioning? (yes/no)

Drug Services Agency Management Questionnaire Outline

A-1: AGENCY PROFILE (FOR AGENCY DIRECTOR/ADMINISTRATOR/MANAGERS)

Agency name

Address

Telephone

Number of years providing service

Hours/days of service

Director's name

Name of the person completing the questionnaire

Client population targeted for service
children
family
youth
    general
    delinquent
    drug and alcohol users
    mentally ill
male adults

     general

     criminals

     drug and alcohol users

     mentally ill

  female adults

     general

     criminals

     drug and alcohol users

     mentally ill

Drug-Using Population (for general human service and drug service agencies)

average total number of clients served at any one time

average number of clients, at any one time, using drugs and/or alcohol

percentage of drug users of the total population of clients served

average number of drug users receiving services who are drug dealers (number of dealers/number of users served)

does your agency maintain a list of those in need of services? (yes/no)

if yes, on average how many addicts are waiting to receive service?

on average, how many weeks of service are provided to each client?

does your agency provide support services to the families of addicts? (yes/no)

does your agency need additional professional staff? (yes/no)

    if yes, which type?

does your agency provide services to female addicts? (yes/no)

    if yes, are at least some of the services separated from the male addicts served?

Number of staff

number of full-time staff

number of part-time staff

number of volunteers

number of staff with professional status (academic degree)

number of staff with paraprofessional status

number of full-time equivalent positions (based on hours of professional, paraprofessional, and volunteer staff)

Staff Functions

number of professional, paraprofessional and volunteer staff involved with:

    direct services

    supervision

    other (list type of service)

Staff education
number of professional, paraprofessional and volunteer staff education level:

did not complete high school

completed high school

university student

university education (with B.A. degree)

university education (with M.A. degree)

university education (with Ph.D.)

other (provide details)

type of higher education

social work

education

sociology

psychology

other (provide details)

Clients Served (check one category)
too many clients in need of service

the number in need can be accommodated with existing resources

too few clients for the resources available

During the last 15 years or less, has your agency had unfilled staff positions because of a lack of qualified personnel available for employment? (yes/no)
If yes, how many unfilled positions have there been; what type of service position has gone unfill.d? (e.g., direct service, supervision, management, etc.)

Staff experience
list the number of staff by their status—in other words, professional, paraprofessional—and the number of years of experience

Is your agency a regional one? (county type service—yes/no)

Which city/town are most of your clients from?

A-2: MANPOWER DEVELOPMENT AND TRAINING

Do staff receive training? (yes/no)
If yes, how effective is the training (e.g., 5 pt. scale: very effective . . . not at all effective)

Who provides the training?
For example, private training institute; university; government experts; experts within the agency, and so on.

Rating of the following training characteristics:
(e.g., 5 pt. scale: very important . . . not at all important):

training relevant to actual practice problems

on-the-job follow-up skills development

available, qualified training staff within the agency

sufficient and available training materials

coordination between training and program staff

training needs assessment

training funds

time-off for staff to attend training

agency support for training purposes

Rating of the following incentives for in-service training participation:
(e.g., 5 pt. scale: very important . . . not at all important):

maintain current job status

obtain promotions

increase salary

obtain a license or certificate

obtain college credits

improve professional skills

improve job performance

provide time-off from the job

Rating of training assistance needed for the following:
(e.g., 5 pt. scale: very much needed . . . not at all needed):

development of a training program

dissemination of relevant training materials

assessing training needs

coordinating training

training staff

development of training materials

training agency trainers

evaluation of training programs

Is someone in the agency responsible for staff development and training? (yes/no)
If yes, how much of the person's time is devoted to this task?

Rating of the following training areas:
(e.g., 5 pt. scale: very important . . . not at all important):

decision making in client services referral and/ placement

working with families as part of a social service/treatment plan

working with involuntary/not cooperative clients

working with broken families

preventive outreach to clients and/or families at risk

client referral and/or placement process

staff supervision

service accountability

identifying and reducing worker stress

workload management

documentation for administrative and/or judicial hearings

psychological and social processes of separation/loss

supplemental services to client and/or family (e.g., day care, home-maker services, etc.)

personal communications

case review and monitoring systems

working with troubled/disturbed clients

management and use of information systems

understanding cultural and social class differences

developing and implementing training for drug service workers

impact of government policies drug services

changing bureaucracy from within

history of the drug problem and philosophy of drug services intervention

working with self-help groups

institutional abuse and neglect of clients

research findings in drug services

drug legislation

community organization

client advocacy

individual counseling

group counseling

family counseling

drug services development

psychosocial development of clients in need of services

team work

interdisciplinary services coordination

working with paraprofessionals and volunteers

supporting the family as part of the treatment process

other (specify)

A-3: AGENCY ASSISTANCE

Rating of need for technical assistance in the following areas:
(e.g., 5 pt. scale: very much needed important . . . not at all needed)

prevention services planning

treatment services planning

prevention services provision

treatment services provision

direct services practice skills development

case management planning and monitoring

methods of case reporting

workload management

management/administration

fiscal budgeting and management

proposal development

services coordination

interpersonal communications

information and dissemination

job definitions and responsibilities

developing working relationships with other human service agencies

other (specify)

Rating of problem areas:
(e.g., 5 pt. scale: very much a problem . . . no problem)

case records contain incomplete or inaccurate information

case records are difficult to review due to:

    unorganized information

    too much information

    subjective information

inconsistencies between workers in the goals they consider for clients in relatively similar cases

case records are misplaced

case records are lost

usual gaps of more than one (1) week in delivery of planned services during inter- or intra-agency transfer of cases

confidentiality of individually identifiable recorded information on clients is often compromised

status information on clients is often inaccurate or outdated

caseworkers and supervisors have difficulty identifying cases that need attention

difficulty providing information to fulfill government reporting requirements

professional staff performing functions that could be handled by paraprofessional staff or volunteers

unacceptable rate of staff absenteeism

staff turnover is higher than 25% during the past year

caseworkers have difficulty in identifying and setting priorities for cases

Rating of research priority areas:
(e.g., 5 pt. scale: very much needed . . . not at all needed)

client needs

the needs of women in the treatment process

family needs and problems

nutrition and eating disorders of addicts

patterns of child care among addicted parents

drug using youth problems and needs

codependency

relation of alcohol and illegal drug use

violence and substance use

service evaluation

the impact of follow-up care (after detoxification)

management and staff organization issues in the work place

patterns of service decision making by workers for clients

(other)

B-1: PERSONAL PROFILE

Name

Address

Primary type of services provided:
emergency intake

treatment

individual counseling

family counseling

group counseling

community organization

residential inpatient treatment

day treatment

training

planning and program development

supervision

management

(other)

Work (time) status

full-time

part-time

volunteer

Employment status

professional

paraprofessional

Job responsibility

direct services

supervision

management/organization

(other)

Education

did not complete high school

completed high school

university student

university education (with B.A. degree)

university education (with M.A. degree)

university education (with Ph.D.)

other (provide details)

If you are a university graduate what was your study concentration:

social work

education

sociology

psychology

other (provide details)

If you have studied at the university, did you have a course or lectures on (yes/no):

drug/alcohol prevention?

drug/alcohol treatment?

drug/alcohol research?

drug/alcohol services management?

If you do not have university education, please report the training/education you have had relevant to your work with drug prevention/treatment

Indicate the total number of cases (active and inactive) you have:

Indicate the average number of active cases you have:

Indicate the average amount of time (hours) that you give each case every two weeks:

Indicate the number years of experience that you have in the following areas:
services

supervision

management/administration

B-2: MANPOWER DEVELOPMENT AND TRAINING (SEE A-2 ITEM INVENTORY)

B-3: AGENCY ASSISTANCE (SEE A-3 ITEM INVENTORY)

Index

About the Authors

RICHARD E. ISRALOWITZ is on the faculty of the Spitzer Department of Social Work, Ben Gurion University, Israel. He is Director of the Regional International Center for Alcohol and Drug Information, an effort sponsored by National Clearinghouse for Alcohol and Drug Information in Washington, DC.

DARWIN TELIAS is a psychiatrist specializing in the field of substance abuse treatment in Israel. He has served as Director of the Drug Treatment Program for Israel Prison Authority and is presently responsible for drug treatment services provided by the regional psychiatric hospital of the Negev located in Beer Sheva.